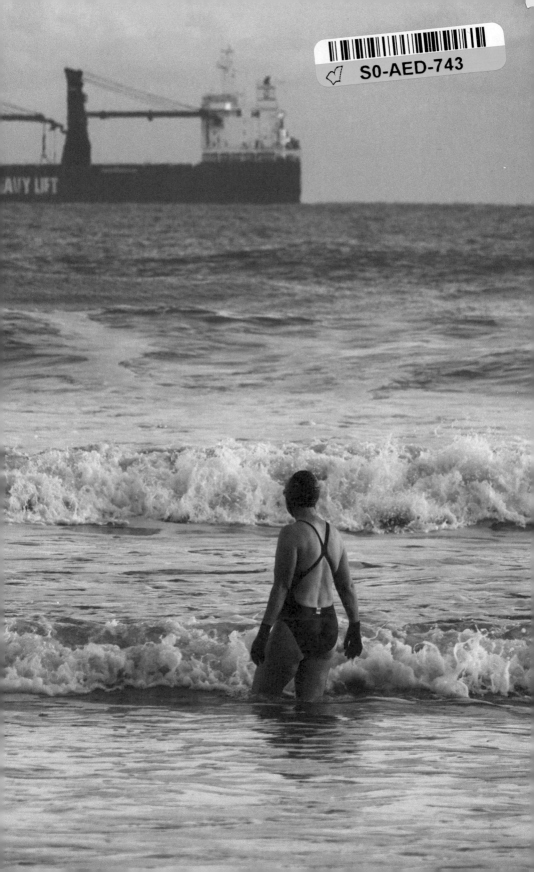

S0-AED-743

WINTER
SWIMMING

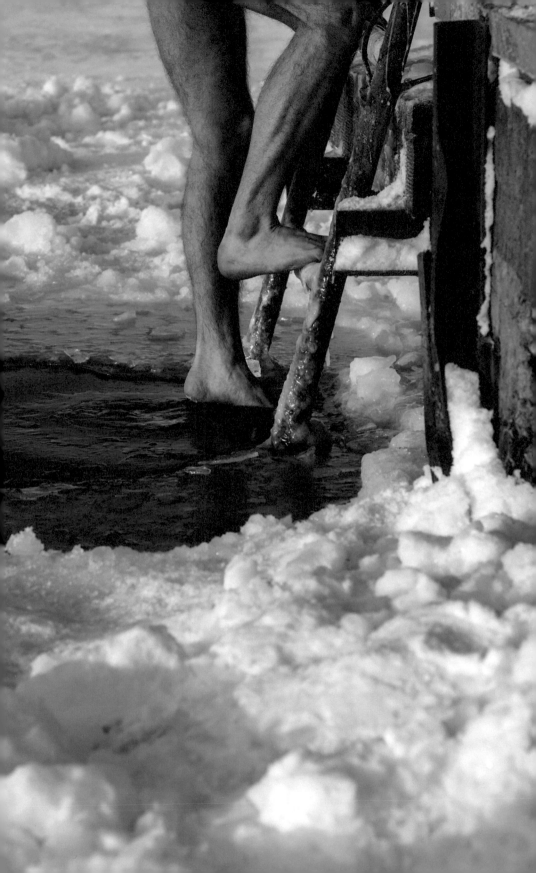

DR SUSANNA SØBERG

WINTER SWIMMING

The Nordic Way Towards a Healthier and Happier Life

Translated from the Danish by
Elizabeth DeNoma

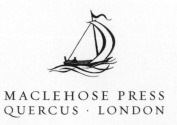

MACLEHOSE PRESS
QUERCUS · LONDON

First published as *Hop i havet – Vinterbadning gør dig sund og glad*
by Grønningen 1 in Copenhagen, Denmark, in 2019

First published in Great Britain in 2022 by

MacLehose Press
An imprint of Quercus Editions Limited
Carmelite House
50 Victoria Embankment
London EC4Y 0DZ

An Hachette UK company

Copyright © Susanna Søberg, 2019
English translation copyright © 2022 by Elizabeth DeNoma
Picture researcher – Cathie Arrington

The moral right of Susanna Søberg to be identified as the author of this work has
been asserted in accordance with the Copyright, Designs and Patents Act, 1988.

Elizabeth DeNoma asserts her moral right to be
identified as the translator of the work.

*Winter swimming is a physically challenging activity and, as with all physical
activities, it carries a risk of personal injury. As such, it may not be suitable for
everyone. If you are unsure whether winter swimming is appropriate for you,
you are advised to consult a doctor before participating.*

All rights reserved. No part of this publication may be reproduced or
transmitted in any form or by any means, electronic or mechanical, including
photocopy, recording, or any information storage and retrieval system,
without permission in writing from the publisher.

A CIP catalogue record for this book is available from the British Library.

ISBN (HB) 978 1 52941 746 3
ISBN (Ebook) 978 1 52941 748 7

10 9 8 7 6 5 4 3 2

Designed by Nick Evans
Printed and bound in China by C & C Offset Printing Co., Ltd.

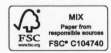

Papers used by Quercus Books are from well-managed forests
and other responsible sources.

CONTENTS

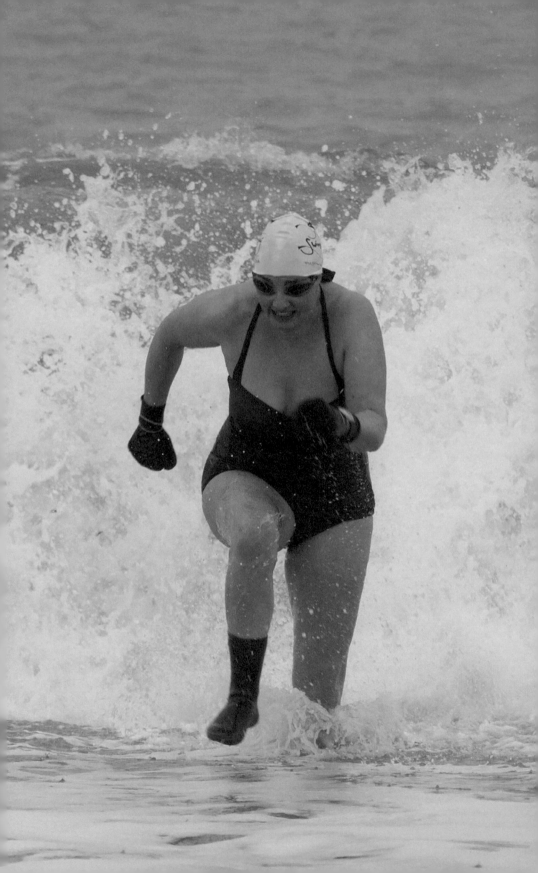

INTRODUCTION

"Life is too exciting to stay neutral"
SUSANNA SØBERG

Disney's superheroine from the blockbuster movie *Frozen* is cool in more ways than one. Leaving aside Elsa's magical ability to build castles from ice and change summer into winter, she is, more than anyone, fond of the cold. And the joy to be found in cold can be recognized by winter swimmers in Denmark and the rest of the world. Cold habituation is nothing supernatural or magical – everyone can achieve the ability to sit or swim in icy water (and even in ice holes) – with a big smile on their face, and to the delight of both body and soul.

There was a time when I found very cold water difficult to endure, but now I've become a winter swimmer and the cold bothers me much less. If a popsicle like me can learn to winter swim, anyone can. It's a question of mindset.

A few years ago, before I became a winter swimmer, my husband and I were walking along the coast of Denmark on an early winter's morning. We noticed a small group of people in bathrobes walking towards the sea. The sun was shining from behind grey-white clouds, and the fog had settled like a wide, white blanket over the blue-black water. There was frost in the air, and it bit our cheeks. "Look, they're going to swim," I said. The men and women went along the jetty and threw off their bathrobes. They were naked. At the end of the jetty they turned, and without hesitation walked step by step down the ladder. The water must have been freezing. "Plop" was the sound as the winter bathers slipped elegantly into the cold water. They had it under control, you could tell. They swam around for a short time and came back up onto the jetty. They smiled and laughed together – wow, what energy!

7

Since then, my husband and I have become winter swimmers and sometimes our children come along too. It's incredibly enjoyable to do together as a family, and afterwards we're all like charged batteries.

"But wait a minute," says the healthy sceptic, "Why would you swim in the winter? It's so unbelievably cold!" The answers to this question lie in the physical, psychological, social and nature aspects of winter swimming. As a researcher, I am glad to know that there's a general interest in what is happening within the body – and a curiosity about what contributes to good health. In this book we will cover many of these topics. The healthy sceptic may gain a perspective on why winter swimming is loved by such a large (and growing) number of people. There's a reason why they're often known as "the happy winter swimmers". And perhaps it will inspire more people to take the plunge.

We all know what it feels like to have a lot on your mind. In my experience, the cold makes you feel great during good times, but even better in bad times. There is nothing – no medication, no other form of exercise – that can shock you out of your head and back into your body like cold water can. In this book, I'm going to explore why.

Many people will be apprehensive and wonder how to get started, or they may believe winter swimming is for the brave few. I've heard people says it's "extreme", or that it takes a lot of strength. But you don't have to be made of something special – like Elsa – or be particularly sporty, for that matter. I advise new winter swimmers to start off in peace and quiet, build up their courage and get used to the cold gradually (habituation). Winter swimming is a social activity which generates happiness, but equally it's a form of stress reduction and a means of self-development in other contexts, too.

This is a guide for new winter swimmers, which may also inspire and challenge experienced swimmers. Winter swimming is something most people can do, and it can be learned. Nevertheless, there are exceptions: winter swimming is not recommended for patients with

---

Page 6: Racing the waves on New Year's Day at Aberystwyth, Wales.

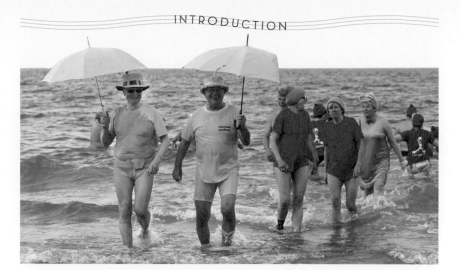

Above: Members of the "Rostock Seehunde" (Rostock Seals) taking part in their traditional end-of-season swim, Rostock-Warnemuende, Germany.

untreated coronary artery disease and/or chest pain (angina pectoris), severe heart arrhythmia or untreated hypertension. If you are in these groups, or are in any doubt, you should first consult your doctor.

In this book I draw on research and the publications of health agencies such as the World Health Organization. I investigate both the immediate and long-term effects of cold-water immersion, although these cannot be dealt with exhaustively in this book as there is still much research to be done. Among other things, we cannot yet know if winter swimming makes us live longer or if there are any long-term risks. These are important questions still to be answered.

Alongside my personal training in winter swimming, I achieved my PhD in Metabolism, specializing in brown fat and winter swimming, from the University of Copenhagen. As a researcher, I feel incredibly lucky to have been able to examine the happiest people in the world!

Some of my own research is also included here, in a survey of 180 adults over the age of eighteen who are not winter swimmers. In addition, I share the experience of the clinical trials from my PhD. The experiments consisted of controlled temperature tests in the laboratory and a randomized controlled experiment, with the introduction of new winter swimmers to the activity from a jetty in

Copenhagen. The subjects had impressive willpower and dedication; it's amazing what the body can do, as long as the brain wants it to. This book gives an insight into the early stages of a scientist's work. The results of my experiments have not yet been made public, and so the material is based on research already available, as well as my experience of carrying out the experiments.

So is winter swimming healthy? This is a good question, and one which I partly highlight in my research, specifically in relation to brown fat. It is an exciting organ, especially if you're a winter swimmer, sleep in the cold or otherwise expose yourself to low temperatures. But, surprisingly, it is barely known about. Brown fat works for your health – it's activated by the cold and generates heat, which leads to increased calorie burning. Brown fat therefore has the potential to treat obesity and type 2 diabetes.

They are also known as "the warm winter swimmers", and many will no doubt nod in recognition of the fact that outdoorsy people don't seem to suffer from the cold. Brown fat bears part of the explanation for that. We may imagine that Elsa, who has fantastic cold habituation, has a lot of brown fat. And who doesn't want to be like Elsa? Winter swimming might be the closest we get to having her superpowers.

Of course, winter swimming is not a new invention. People have been taking to cold water since time immemorial, but for various reasons it's now having a renaissance.

Allow me to start by inviting you on a journey in time to the fourth century BCE, when the first anecdotes about cold water and health began to be told. Then we'll board a ship with the famous Scottish doctor James Currie . . .

Opposite: Taking an icy dip on Christmas Day builds a healthy appetite!

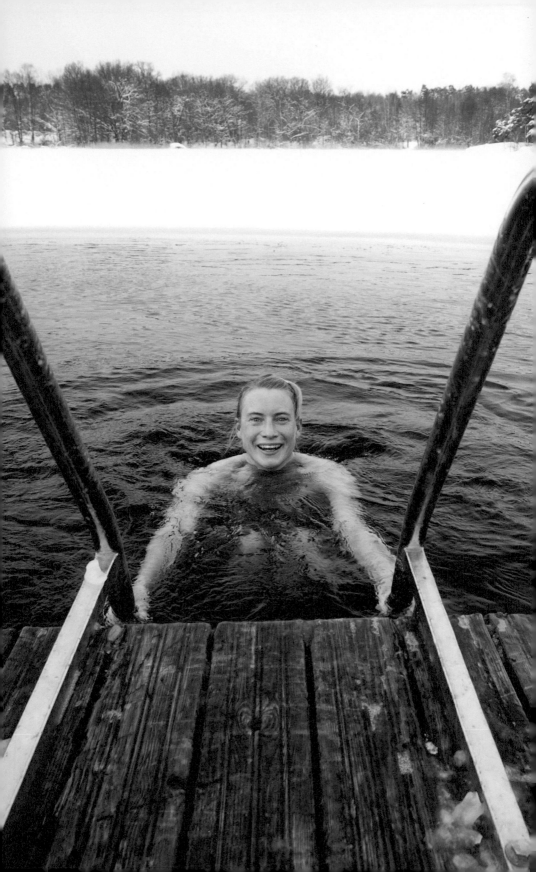

CHAPTER 1

WINTER SWIMMING THROUGH TIME

"Nothing burns the skin like cold!"
GEORGE R.R. MARTIN
Author of *A Song of Ice and Fire*

VOL. LXXV.—No. 1929
Week Ending February 21, 1914
PRICE TEN CENTS

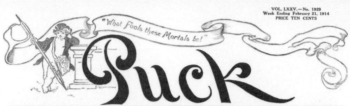

"What Fools these Mortals be!"

Puck

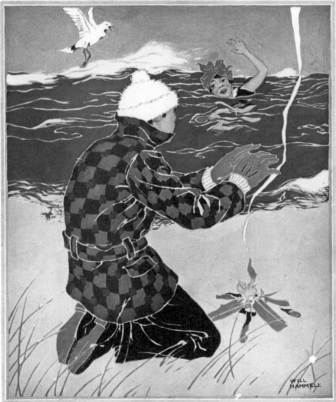

A MID-WINTER MARTYR.

THE CHAP WHOSE FIANCÉE IS AN ALL-YEAR BATHING-GIRL.

1

Throughout history, cold water has been a friend and a foe to humanity, with both beneficial and harmful effects. That is to say, it's nothing new for people to be interested in the effects of cold water.

According to Hippocrates, who lived around the fourth century BCE, water therapy reduced violence; and for sixty years in the eighteenth and nineteenth centuries, Thomas Jefferson swore by taking a cold foot bath every morning to maintain his good health.

But to a large extent, interest in the effects of cold water on well-being and health was based on anecdotal evidence. It was simply assumed that there were a number of health benefits as a consequence of specific physiological reactions and the biochemical environment occurring in our bodies upon exposure to cold water. It was also believed, even before the advent of modern science, that acute physiological changes occurred upon initial exposure to cold water, while repetition elicited physiological adaptive responses and a number of positive long-term health benefits.

The dawn of science

In the Middle Ages, people were generally not taught to swim, even if they lived near to the water or depended on it for their livelihoods.

The return to swimming in Western Europe began only in the sixteenth century. In 1538 Nikolaus Wynmann, a German professor of languages, wrote the first book on swimming, *The Swimmer* or *A Dialogue on the Art of Swimming*. His intention was to persuade more people to learn to swim, to reduce the number of drowning accidents. This foreshadowed modern science's more pragmatic approach to being in water.

In December 1790, the Scottish physician James Currie witnessed the drowning of the crew of a capsized American sailing ship. The sea was 5°C (41°F), and the crew perished from hypothermia. The event made a great impression on Currie and led him to undertake the first experiments to measure the effect of cold water on humans. He became the first to discover that cold water acts as a stimulus on the central nervous system. Currie was also behind

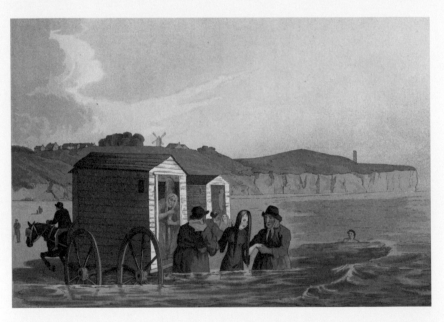

Above: Sea bathing at Scarborough, as depicted in *The Costume of Yorkshire* by George Walker in 1814.

Page 14: Cover of *Puck* magazine from February 1914 depicting "The chap whose fiancée is an all-year bathing-girl". Illustration by Will Hammell.

the first scientific reports on the healing properties of cold water; for example, he investigated whether the cold could cure fever. In 1797, on a ship off Jamaica, he developed a fever and recorded the following experience:

> September 9th, having given the necessary directions, about three o'clock in the afternoon I stripped off all my clothes, and threw a sea-cloak loosely about me till I got upon deck, when the cloak also was laid aside: three buckets full of cold salt water were then thrown at once on me; the shock was great, but I felt immediate relief. The headache and other pains instantly abated, and a fine glow and diaphoresis succeeded. Towards evening, however, the febrile symptoms threatened a return, and I had again recourse to the same method, as before, with the same good effect. I now took food with an appetite, and for the first time had a sound night's rest.
>
> James Currie, 1797

It was later deemed inappropriate and decidedly contraindicated to treat fever patients with cold water. Aside from conducting experiments on fever, Currie carried out temperature experiments throughout his life and documented many other effects of cold water, effects which today we consider positive.

Sea swimming then and now

As early as 1750, the governments of several northern European coastal nations made formal recommendations about swimming in seawater – as well as drinking it – to treat a number of diseases. (Today we know that seawater has a high salt content and can cause vomiting when drunk, due to the osmotic effect of salt and water in the gut. That must have been an interesting experience, and one would hope the recommendation was quickly revoked.) Winter was considered the best time to swim. Sea swimming reached the peak of its popularity

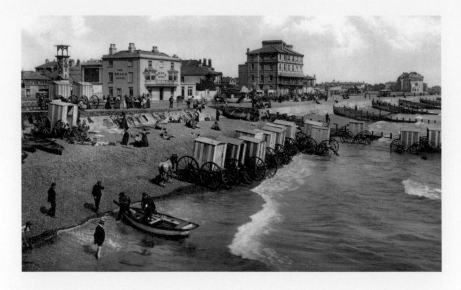

Above: Bathing machines at the edge of the water in Bognor Regis, England, c. 1890.

in the late eighteenth century with the development of the bathing suit and "bathing machine". Bathing machines were designed to give women in particular the opportunity to change into swimwear in a private space, and then go directly into the water. The small wooden bathing machines had wheels, a roof and doors at both ends of the house. Since then, bathhouses have evolved into more stationary structures on the beach, and today are often to be found painted in bright, beautiful colours. They still function as changing rooms, now for both men and women.

It was also in the eighteenth century that entire communities and seaside resorts were founded on the basis that sea swimming brought health benefits. The risk of drowning accidents led to the introduction of "beach rescue" and lifeguards. The modern trend of open sea swimming may well have been established on 3 May 1810, when Lord Byron swam several kilometres along the Dardanelles over Hellespont. Even today, some two hundred years later, swimmers compete to achieve Byron's feat in ice-cold water. In general, there is a marked and increasing interest in open cold-water swimming, with ice-swimming

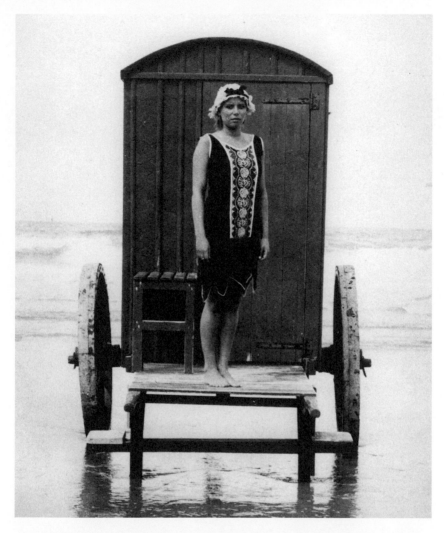

Above: Woman and bathing machine on the North Sea island of Borkum, Germany, January 1914.

competitions, marathon swimming and triathlons. General winter swimming or winter dipping is common today among all ages, and should be seen as a non-competitive activity. Instead, it serves another purpose: winter swimming and dipping encourages inner focus, meditation and enhanced well-being, as well as being a social activity. With more winter swimmers and different cold-water practices, there

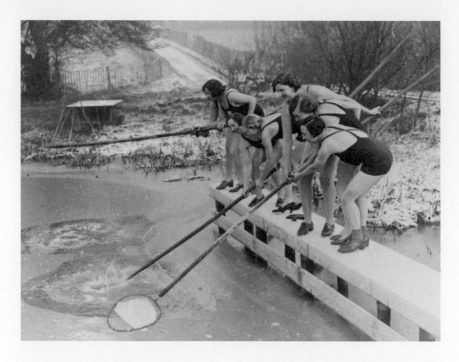

is also an increased interest in research into the physiological and psychological benefits associated with being in cold water.

Many people think of winter swimming as taking a mental break, alongside reaping some health benefits and giving oneself a sense of empowerment. In a world dominated by technology our brains are online almost 24/7, and so it is a gift for body and soul to give ourselves a respite. This respite could consist of exercise, but it could also be a more extreme physical activity such as winter swimming, with a sauna visit to enhance the experience of Zen and calmness afterwards. In this book I will take you through the practice and theory as well as the stories, and endeavour to unfold how this is all connected.

Above: Regulars clear the ice at Kenwood Ladies' Pond, Hampstead Heath, London, December 1935.

Opposite: The Polar Bear Club of Milwaukee takes a dip in Lake Michigan on New Year's Day 1972. (The photographer wore a wetsuit.)

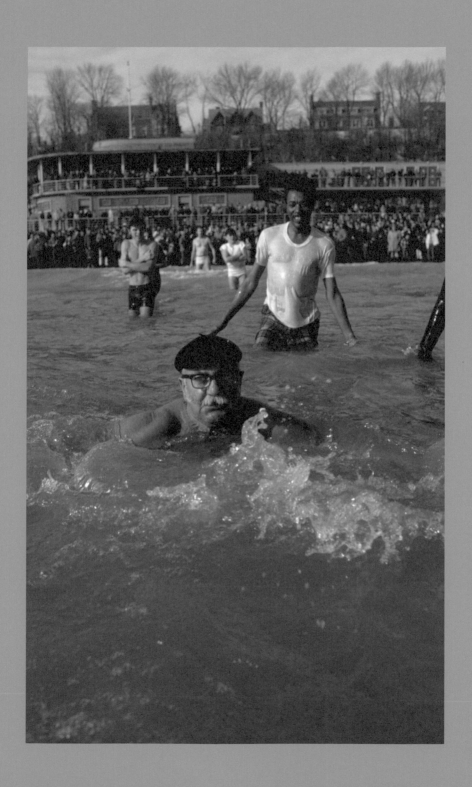

CHAPTER 2

WHY SWIM IN THE WINTER?

"Let us love winter,
for it is the spring of genius"
PIETRO ARETINO
Italian author and politician

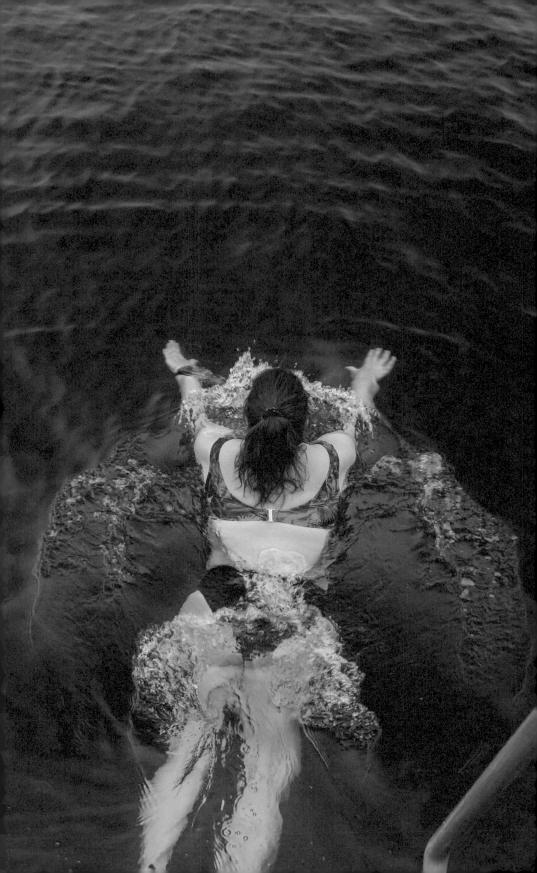

2

Other than Singapore, Denmark, where I live, has the longest coastline in the world relative to its total area, and nowhere in Denmark is more than fifty kilometres away from the sea. With many large lakes as well, we're very lucky to have such easy access to water.

Many winter swimmers live close to the water, already have an innate appreciation of this ever-changing element and enjoy communing with nature. With water so accessible, it is neither expensive nor very time consuming to become a winter swimmer.

More and more people are recognizing the positive effects of cold water, and the waiting lists for winter swimming clubs have grown to be years long. Winter swimming seems to provide something that we long for in our societies, perhaps as a counterweight to other habits that we're trying to distance ourselves from, whether it's an overconsumption of beer, too much time at the computer or excess snacking. During the Covid-pandemic lockdowns, there was an increased uptake of winter swimming, as documented all over social media. People who until then may not have got further than thinking about becoming a winter swimmer now jumped into their new healthy habit for the thrill and laughs it would give them and a few chosen friends. Perhaps a niche activity some years ago, during the last few years winter swimming has grown to become almost mainstream. It has certainly become a way of challenging oneself, as well as a health and wellness trend, and something real that gets us away from technology.

Inner peace and abundance

The feeling of intoxication, the breathing and getting in touch with nature seem to be universally soothing and satisfying. The winter swimmers I spoke to, both the old-hands and the newbies, describe a feeling of being able to shift their focus away from negative thoughts to concentrating solely on what is happening in the moment: descending step by step into the icy water, without thinking, and feeling nature so intimately that it's as if you're a part of it all. And all the while your problems seem to recede.

The shock of the cold water demands full attention from body and mind to survive, because the mind interprets cold-water swimming as a life-threatening situation. The experience is generally described as a kind of positive shock, a moment of reset, in which your brain gets a kick-start of energy and you're ready to face whatever comes your way. The positive energy is most likely due to an increase of the neurotransmitters dopamine and serotonin. These control mood and mental balance. Scientists are not sure how antidepressant medicine works, as it is difficult to measure neurotransmission live in the human brain. However, it is believed that the medicine increases the levels of certain neurotransmitters, such as serotonin, noradrenalin and dopamine, which are linked to mood and emotion. We assume that the effect of cold water does the same, and an increase in dopamine would explain the positive effects on mental health, mood and energy described by winter swimmers. The outcome is an increased inner power that can be used in self-development and channelled into all kinds of other activities.

Page 24: Winter swimming in Copenhagen, Denmark.

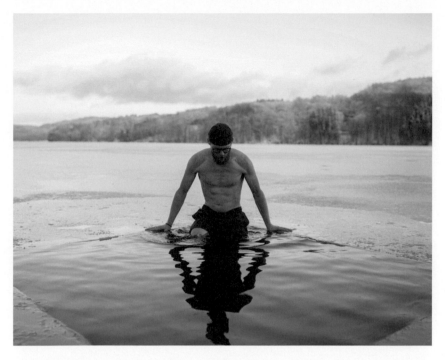

Above: The shock of cold water demands full attention because the mind interprets cold-water swimming as a life-threatening situation.

A winter swimmer in one of my studies came to the laboratory for a first test after three months of winter swimming. We asked him if he liked winter swimming so far. His face lit up and, smiling, he described the effect as increased "patience" and a sense of "ease". He further described how he washed away his road rage with his morning swims, and was happy to let other drivers pass on his way to work. Others in the study described having increased focus at work, while still others experienced more calm and better sleep. There are many different effects, depending on the motivation for taking up winter swimming in the first place. When asked, our subjects with chronic pain claimed the water reduced their discomfort, while those without pain reported increased happiness, better health and sleep, and reduced stress. These observations are in line with results from a worldwide questionnaire of 482 sauna-bathers by Hussain J.N. et al., 2016. In this study, both men and women answered that the key reasons they used saunas included relaxation/stress reduction, pain relief and socializing. In Nordic countries, combining winter swimming and hot saunas is becoming increasingly popular. Despite the differences in their answers, most people responded that the contact with nature gave them greater energy and a feeling of inner peace.

For many people, open-water swimming is about more than just getting into the water. It's also an experience of nature: the smell of seawater, the silence, the birds on the sea and, not least, following the changing seasons.

A sense of the seasons

From the shore, you can observe from day to day the range of seasonal conditions, from the hottest day in summer to the coldest in winter. In Denmark we are not blessed with mountains, waterfalls, volcanoes or

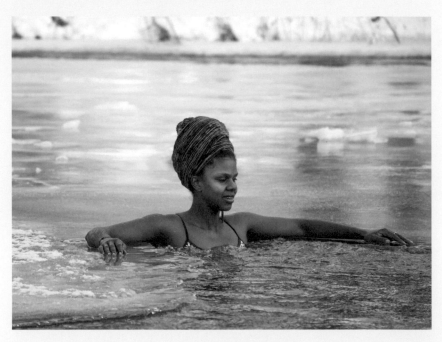

Above: Winter swimmers describe a feeling of being able to shift their focus away from negative thoughts to concentrating solely on the moment.

similar dramatic and dominant natural features rising high above sea level. Denmark is a flat country, with what we ourselves often refer to as boring nature. But we do have something that's worth showcasing – the beautiful changing seasons and lots of water, to which we have ample access and can easily enjoy.

When winter comes, we don't usually have the opportunity to strap on skis for cross-country or slalom skiing, but we can get an energy boost and a burst of joy throughout the winter months, from October to the end of April. And for those winter swimmers who have access to a sauna, and have the opportunity to feel both cold and heat throughout the season, it's even more exhilarating. The interaction between heat and cold, the hormones and nerve signals resulting from the stimuli, is likely to have a positive effect on people prone to winter depression, or seasonal affective disorder (SAD). People I have spoken to in my research who suffer from SAD say that winter swimming has changed their view of winter from a dark and dull season to a happy and exciting one. They no longer abhor winter, and even share the advice that "kick-starting your day with winter swimming is even better than morning coffee". I wouldn't exchange my morning coffee for it, but the advice makes sense. The effect of winter swimming on SAD or depression has not yet been scientifically explored, but it will be before long, I am sure.

Nature is surprising. We know the colours and smells of spring and warmer weather, but the change in season you feel in the water is something special. The physiological effects of the cold take you into your body and out of your brain, and immediately demand your presence. I have learned that every swim is different, every season is a new experience in nature, and it never gets boring.

The "cold-shock response"

In the Nordic countries we have practised winter swimming for centuries, although mostly the older generations. Today, the younger generations are following along, which probably makes winter swimming the most unisex and uni-age form of activity you can undertake. Winter swimming. Winter bathing. Cold-water swimming. Ice swimming. Wild swimming or winter dipping. It's not overly important what we call it. The formula is simple: take off your clothes, get into the icy water, feel the stinging cold on your skin – brrrrrr – get out of the water – feel the rush throughout your body – aaaaaaaaaahhhhh – that feeling!

After our dip or swim, we may be surprised to feel warm and happy. So what really happens to us? The effects are not as concrete or easy to describe as the action itself. As soon as I feel the cold water again, I certainly recognize it and my body remembers it right away. But when I get out of the water, the remarkably intense physical sensation disappears, and is overtaken by a feeling of calmness, joy and warmth. However wonderful, it's still a difficult feeling to grasp or convey. All I can suggest is that you try it yourself and determine if it's right for you. There might be a number of barriers. Winter swimming is cold, yes, and for many that's probably one of the most off-putting factors. Avoiding the cold is normal in our modern society, but exposing yourself to the cold is the way to overcome it.

During my research we trained fifteen overweight pre-diabetic subjects in winter swimming. None of them had ever tried winter swimming or cold showers. The first weeks of winter swimming were tough, but the team and I were on hand and even went in the water with the subjects. It was a great success. My experience is that you need support with at least one or two swim-buddies who will keep you motivated on those cold days.

When you get through the first winter season, you'll have conquered the mental and physical challenge it requires. Then during the summer you can rejoice that your body is smart enough to remember your earlier ordeals. This is due to a building resilience, also known as cold

---

Opposite: Winter bathers emerge from the icy Zweigkanal after a six-kilometre (four-mile) run – a New Year tradition in Letter, Seelze, Germany.

habituation. Studies in humans measuring the respiratory rate, blood pressure, heart rate and norepinephrine (a chemical functioning as both a hormone and a neurotransmitter) upon cold-water immersion before the first and second winter swimming season show that the cold-shock response is lower before the second season. This means that you don't have to start over from scratch the next winter. The human body is incredible! Getting through the first season is an achievement; your winter swimming will never get tougher than that. You can transfer that will and perseverance to other goals: to lose weight, for example, or to start training or running – you will access the same stores of willpower when it's hard to put on your running shoes and get out of the door. If you have succeeded in becoming a winter swimmer, you have already proven to yourself that you can do anything you put your mind and heart to.

Of course, there are many activities one can take up in nature, but the advantage of winter swimming is that the cold-shock response forces you completely into the moment – you are present, it's cold, you breathe, you feel fresh air and the stinging cold throughout your body. You're forced into the presence of nature, which delivers just

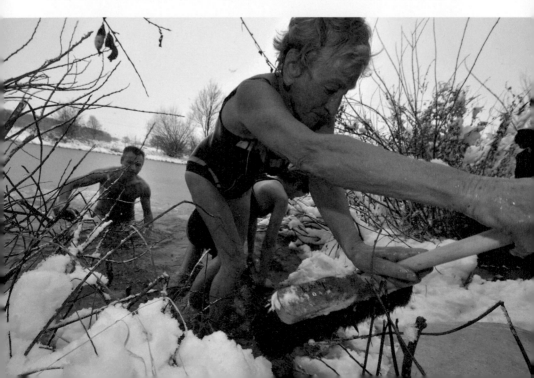

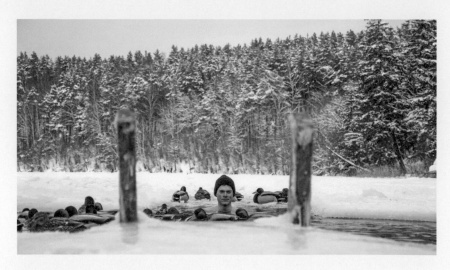

Above: Nature is honest and sincere.

what it intended. There is nothing disingenuous about the effect of cold water. Nature is honest and sincere.

The pace of nature is slow motion

Swimming in cold water goes back a long way in human history, and its effects have not changed. Contrary to the rapid pace of our society and the technological innovations that challenge us in the present, and will perhaps more so in the future, nature moves in slow motion. Some people would like to stop, reflect, and simply feel and take a breath. Today much of our work is sedentary and fast-paced, and plenty of people will nod in recognition at the notion of "sensory overload" after a hard day. The body, on the other hand, has not been doing nearly as much. If the body could talk, it would probably ask you to wake it up and take a walk, run, exercise or swim – and give the brain a rest. This is something swimming in cold water provides – an activation of the body, and respite for the brain.

The motivation of winter swimmers

For busy people in the Nordic countries, winter swimming and saunas are ideal forms of self-pampering and don't take up too much time. And for everyone they can mean something completely different. Some people become hooked on the rush of joy they experience encountering cold water. For others it means freedom and cosiness, hardening against the cold, being part of a competition or mastering a personal challenge. Others do it for health reasons, as they feel healthier in general when they swim and sweat afterwards in the sauna. The motivations are often related to the variety of effects that cold water and a hot sauna can have on the body and brain. In this way, the sea can be a place for development, or for changing your "swim-character", if you like. Being a winter swimmer or "dipper" has a completely different motivation from being an ice swimmer competing in tournaments.

Winter swimming is third on the list of things Danes love, right after chocolate. Why do you think it's so popular?

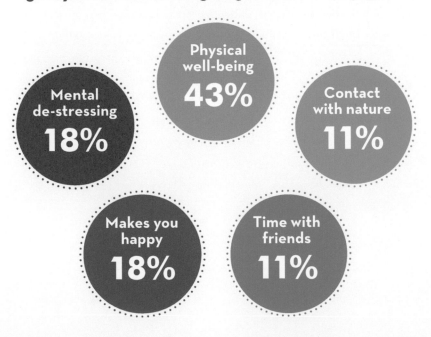

The author asked non-winter swimmers what they thought the attraction was.

You can develop your winter swimming by increasing the time you spend in the water, alongside increasing your familiarization with the water and cold habituation. Whether staying one, two, three or more minutes in cold water increases the health benefits or risks is not known. Furthermore, we do not yet know the health benefits or risks of winter swimming over many years, even if swimmers themselves are convinced that the icy water is beneficial. On the jetty many myths abound that I imagined had been dispensed with long ago, such as "Don't swim right after a meal, you could drown." Many children have waited for hours on the beach because of this admonition, but there is no scientific evidence for it. Or for swimming naked, because the extra sunlight is supposed to be healthier for the body. It is doubtful that a little swimsuit makes any difference.

In the past decade, research has provided some answers – and they need to see the light of day, so that winter swimming does not remain shrouded in unscientific health claims. This information may also give anyone who is not yet a cold-water swimmer the best possible basis to determine for themselves whether it will become their next project.

In this book you will learn something new about your body and its response to different temperatures. You will also become more familiar with a very specialized and delimited type of adipose tissue with particular functions, which is itself an independent organ. You probably don't know much about brown fat yet, but scientifically it provides all the motivation you need to take a winter swim. For me, as a researcher, this fully justifies the enormous popularity of winter swimming.

Opposite: The tranquility of Nature's mirror.

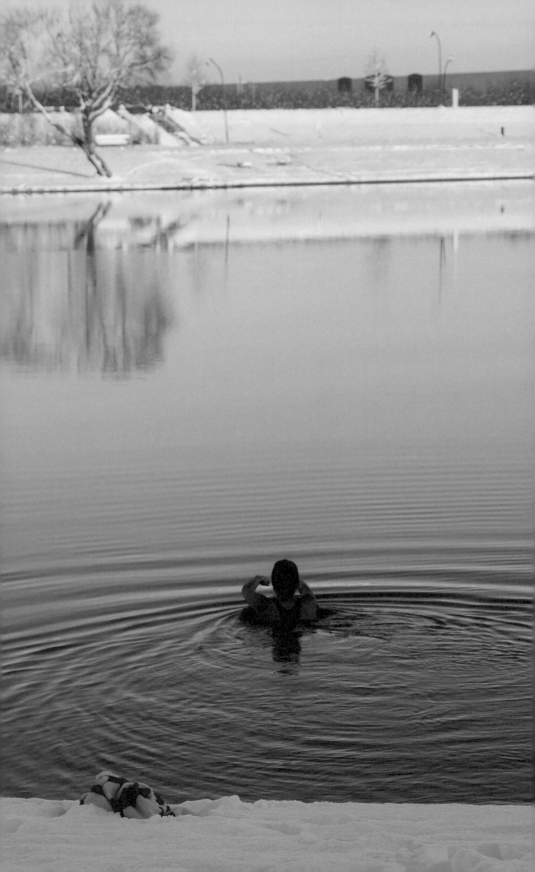

CHAPTER 3

THE WHERE, HOW AND WHEN OF WINTER SWIMMING

"Water is to me, I confess, a phenomenon which continually awakens new feelings of wonder as often as I view it"

MICHAEL FARADAY
Physicist and chemist

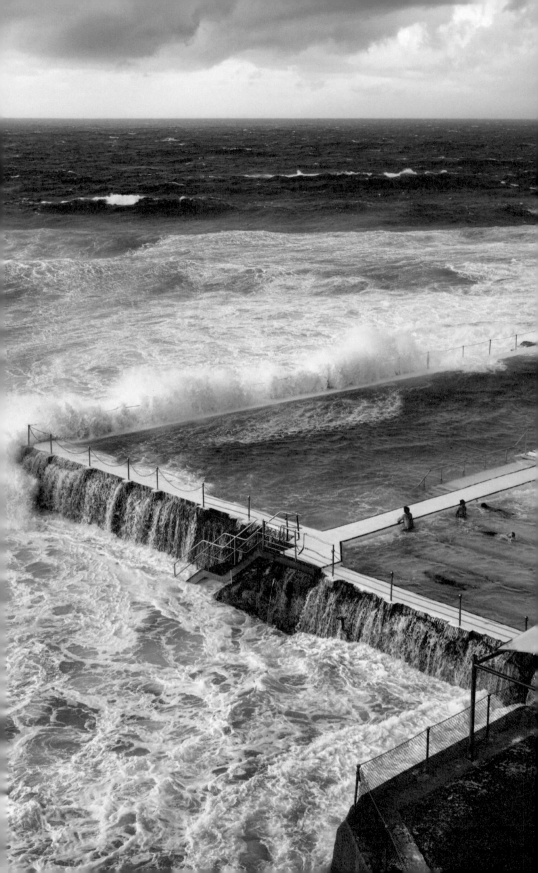

3

When I began my research into brown fat and temperature variation, I imagined that winter swimming took place primarily in colder climates such as Scandinavia, maybe in Russia and Canada, too. However, I soon learned otherwise; winter swimming happens all over the world, in great style, and wherever cold temperatures can be found.

Winter swimming is simply immersion in cold water that happens during the winter season, typically outdoors in the open sea or lakes, or in unheated pools. In colder countries, it can be synonymous with ice swimming, where in order to be able to swim in the water you either have to break the ice or enter the water where a small waterfall or inlet with running water prevents ice from forming. Each singular environment determines how winter swimming is practised in the individual countries and regions.

Winter swimming around the world
In Finland, northern Russia, Norway, Sweden, Estonia, Latvia and Lithuania, winter swimming has been associated with the long-standing

sauna tradition for many years. Denmark has a long history of winter swimming but a relatively short tradition of combining it with a sauna. Ice swimming has always been very popular in Estonia and Finland, and Finns, in particular, are known for their fantastic sauna tradition. To date, the popularity of taking a sauna in Finland is unrivalled.

In Australia, the oldest winter swimming club in the country is reportedly the Bronte Splashers, in Sydney, founded in 1921, with the Bondi Icebergs Club following in 1929, set up by a group of lifeguards who wanted to keep up their training in the winter months. Winter swimming has now become competitive, with many clubs together forming the Winter Swimming Association, and thousands of swimmers competing during the winter months.

In the UK and Ireland, there's been an increase in the number of winter swimmers at the most sought-after locations such as the Serpentine in Hyde Park and Highgate Ponds in London. In London and elsewhere there are freshwater lidos, the largest being Tooting Bec Lido in south-west London, almost twice the length of an Olympic pool at 100 yards (91.44 metres), and competitions take place here even on Christmas Day and New Year's Day. And of course there is the entire coastline, where groups of winter swimmers have been especially active throughout the Covid pandemic. The "Forty Foot" promontory in the south of Dublin Bay has been a popular swimming spot for 250 years.

France, too, is blessed with a long coastline of more than a thousand kilometres (600 miles), and the inland waterways include several natural and artificial lakes, the largest being Lake Bourget and Lake Annecy at the western edge of the Alps. Besides the natural lakes there are also several ponds and lagoons along the Atlantic coast in

---

Page 38: The famous salt-water swimming pool at Bondi, Sydney, Australia – home to the Bondi Icebergs Winter Swimming Club, founded in 1929.

Opposite: Swimming in December at Sandycove Forty Foot bathing area, Dun Laoghaire, a coastal suburb of Dublin, Ireland.

the Landes region and the Mediterranean coast in Languedoc. In Paris, swimming in the waterways is not legal, but nonetheless, during the hot weather a few years ago, the Laboratoire des Baignades Urbaines Expérimentales (Laboratory of Experimental Urban Swimming) was founded, bringing people together in collective swims in the city centre. This in turn led to the formation of an unofficial Paris Wild Swimming Group.

Belgium's winter swimmers use the pools, lakes and rivers all year round, with good spots in Bruges, Boom, Deurne Dendermonde, Wachtebeke, Theux and Huy. The most famous competitions take place at the Meuse river every Sunday in February, and have done since 1963. In the Netherlands and Belgium, winter swimming has been growing in popularity since Deventer opened the first Walrus Club in 2013, and thereafter also in Zutphen, Leeuwarden and Rotterdam. Their members swim in Ijssel, Bergel near Zutphen, de Grote Wielen near Leeuwarden and Waal. The lakes in Germany are popular winter swimming destinations, and especially around Berlin. The Wöhrsee, a lake in Burghausen, hosts an event organized by the International Ice Swimming Assocation.

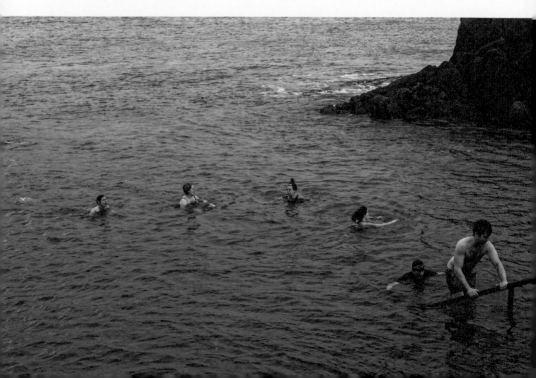

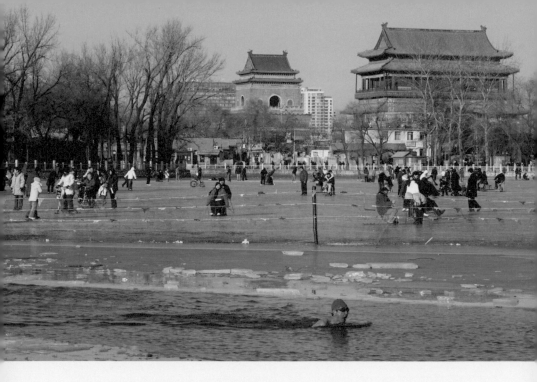

Above: Winter swimming, Houhai, Beijing, China.

On the other side of the world, in China, there are around 140 winter swimming organizations, with more that 200,000 members. The youngest are about ten years old and the oldest well over eighty. In Beijing there are the lakes Shichahai, and those in Yuyuantan park, and in Harbin, northern China, the Songhua river attracts many ice swimmers. In Jinan, at the annual winter swimming festival, the main event involves swimming 300 metres (330 yards) across Daming Lake. In Taiyuan, the air temperature often falls below 10°C (50°F) in the winter, and hundreds of men and women swim every day in the Fen river. Also in north-eastern China, in the coastal city of Dalian, many swim in the lake in winter, but the beaches of the city are even more popular.

In Russia and other Eastern European countries, where Orthodox Christianity is the most widespread religion, ice swimming is associated with the celebration of Epiphany on 19 January. Cruciform-shaped holes are cut into the ice on lakes, rivers and other areas of frozen water. At around midnight a ritual begins in which a

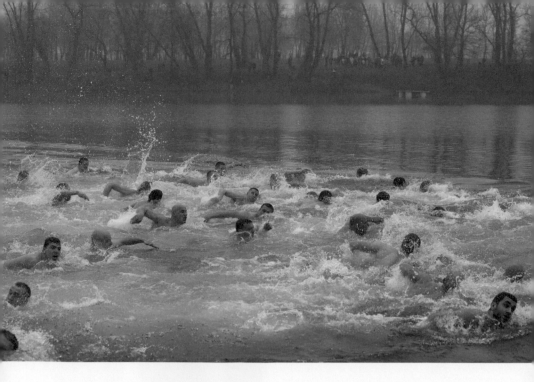

Above: Traditional ice swimming in Belgrade.

priest recites a prayer, and people then immerse themselves into the water three times. There is a popular belief associated with the cold water, namely that it cleanses away our sins. The ritual does not originate in the Russian Orthodox Church, however, but rather from folk tradition. The same traditions are observed also out in Belarus, Ukraine, Kazakhstan and Kyrgyzstan. Bulgaria, Romania, Serbia and Montenegro also celebrate Epiphany in a similar way, although here priests throw wooden crosses into the water, which the swimmers then retrieve. Whoever brings back the crosses will be freed from evil spirits and blessed with good health for the year to come.

In the USA, there are a number of so-called Polar Bear Clubs, where people swim outdoors in the winter and in sponsored events to raise money for charity. The oldest ice swimming club in the United States is thought to be the Coney Island Polar Bear Club in New York, founded in 1903, running events in the Atlantic every Sunday from November to April.

It's quite fascinating that winter swimming is practised in so many different places in the world. Seeing how widespread it is might inspire winter-swimming excursions in other countries too.

Ice swimming and ice bathing

In the Nordic countries, swimming between October and May is considered "winter swimming". Cold exposure can also mean sitting or rolling in the snow, which is quite popular in Finland. Other, more alternative ways to get into cold water include placing a large tub in beautiful surroundings, the forest, for example, filling it with water and large blocks of ice, and taking turns jumping into the tub with your friends. This is known as "ice bathing". Others swim through broken ice, when the temperature is low enough – "ice swimming". What both approaches share is that they take place in nature.

How long and how often?

Practising winter swimming by taking a dip in ice-cold water three to five times, for a few seconds or up to several minutes, between sauna sessions of five to fifteen minutes, is certainly a big challenge for you and your body. Many people practise winter swimming as a thermal interchange between hot and cold.

Active winter swimmers in Denmark's clubs swim on average twice a week. As with other sports, you can claim to be a winter swimmer when you do it with regularity. A "Viking" is not something you are, but something you become. It is therefore important to persevere and continue with your winter-swimming mission, even if you feel a change in the weather and it has become extra cold. It certainly requires discipline, but that is also the point – to exercise self-control and simultaneously to let go when you hit the cold water. It is a mental and physical challenge, but if you can overcome it, you will have cognitive rewards, because you will have pushed your mental limits several times during the process. Overcoming that mental barrier gives you the resources and confidence to overcome other barriers, either new or long-term, because now you know you can push for

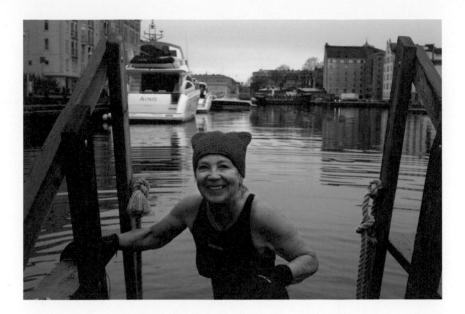

Above: Katajanokka Guest Harbour, Helsinki, Finland.

new goals. Prepare to take a journey of self-control. Forget the hustle and bustle of everyday life and treat yourself to a cold respite. You need to train for this as you would for any other form of physical achievement. So we'd better get started!

The best time of year to start

"It's best to just keep on swimming after summer. Then you'll get used to the cold water more gradually." Many future winter swimmers are likely hear to this when they ask advice from experienced swim "Vikings". This is a rather interesting exhortation, because why wouldn't it be just as easy to start in the winter? There are no statistics to show how many continue winter swimming after starting in summer or winter respectively. However, we can compare ways in which you might start in summer to how you might in winter, to see how the experiences may differ in each season. Either way, it is a good idea to plan with a couple of other people. Swimming in small groups provides both security and safety – and it's simply more fun.

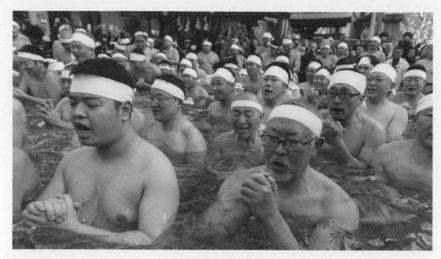

Above: Worshippers at the annual midwinter *Kanchu-Suiyoku* purification ceremony at the Teppozu Inari Shrine, Tokyo, Japan. The pool contains large blocks of ice.

An advantage to continuing to swim after summer ends is that your work is more about maintaining your positive routine, and less about temperature. Building good habits takes time, and is most successfully achieved when you've already got the momentum going. If you've been swimming in the summer, just keep going, even when the calendar turns to September – and be stubborn! You won't experience quite as much of an endorphin kick as if you had started in the winter, but it's a more gentle beginning to simply extend your summer swimming and get used to the cold bit by bit.

At the edge of the cold water

In terms of our perception of water temperature, there is a threshold of around 15°C (60°F), after which we experience the water as freezing cold. One day in September you will be surprised by how the water went from being pleasant to biting and stinging. The gasping reflex is activated, and you suddenly suck in air for the first twenty to thirty seconds. Rejoice, despite the cold! When the water temperature is below 15°C (60°F) the skin's cold receptors will signal to the brain to activate your fight-or-flight response: the cold-shock response.

A cascade of hormones and neurotransmitters puts your body on alert, and this is followed by a rush of joy. By the time the calendar reaches October, it may be called "winter swimming", and you can celebrate that you are already up and running. It makes sense that experienced winter swimmers recommend this model for those new to the sport, as it is a smooth and safe transition to the lower temperatures. It is also recommended for the elderly or those with heart conditions, and only when cold-water swimming is approved by a practitioner. The gradual habituation to the cold water is easier and less stressful on the cardiovascular system. Cold water causes arrhythmia to the heart, and this is much more pronounced in – and potentially dangerous to – people with (known or unknown) heart conditions, especially if starting off in the coldest months. Adaptation is also possible by training with cold showers (see Chapter 6, Cold Acclimatization).

Starting in winter

Some feel that the temperature difference between water and air is too great in autumn. Young novice winter swimmers from my studies felt that starting in winter was preferable because water and air are about the same temperature. If you feel that way, it can be an advantage to start in winter.

In winter the air cools the body before it enters the water, making the water less shockingly cold. This is due to the activation of cold receptors in the skin as you are walking towards the water. This signalling to the brain will increase norepinephrine and endorphins, and vasoconstriction of the peripheral vessels will occur in the skin, numbing the skin before you enter the water. This results in diminished cold perception and a reduced threat to the standard body temperature. In Denmark when the air in February gets warmer, the body cools more slowly in the air, while the water is still as icy cold as it was in January. The temperature differential between the body's surface and the water becomes greater and it may feel as though the water has got colder, despite warmer weather.

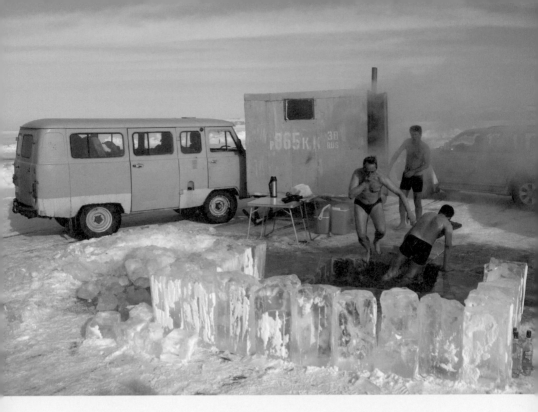

Above: Ice-hole swimming on Lake Baikal, Olkhon Island, Siberia, Russia.

All year round

If you are healthy and have no heart condition, bear in mind that you can start at any time of the year. Winter swimming, working out in the gym, running – or anything else that contributes to your good health but requires effort – are impulses that should be acted on while you're motivated. No matter how good your intentions, they are likely to lose momentum if you do nothing with them. So, if you have an idea or a desire to do something positive for your health, don't wait for the perfect time – it might never come. Carpe diem, seize the day! If you want to try cold-water swimming, it would be a shame to wait and risk it not happening at all, and if you start now, you'll see results a day earlier than if you start tomorrow!

Water and air temperature

In our latest research project with winter swimmers, the participants measured water and air temperatures each time they went out for a

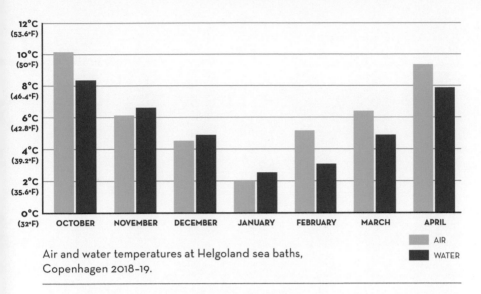

Air and water temperatures at Helgoland sea baths,
Copenhagen 2018–19.

swim, three times a week. This way, we attained a unique data set, with water and air temperatures measured multiple times every day for an entire winter swimming season in Copenhagen (see diagram above). In Denmark the difference between air and water temperatures is greatest in October, February, March and April. In these months your body needs to reacclimatize to the cold-shock response – a new phase of adaptation and thrills. In fact these changes will occur through the winter-swimming season, depending on air temperature, water temperature and wind on any given day. We must honour our changing seasons and beautiful nature in Denmark – it's certainly never boring. Luckily, this is also true for other countries in the world with changing seasons.

It is an intense experience to start swimming in the winter months. Many describe it as very challenging to undertake the icy plunge repeatedly, and it is not only mentally demanding but physically too. Water between 2 and 4°C (36 and 39°F) is very cold, and activates the body's pain receptors – you get the cold-shock response. The body wants to escape, but in order to do so and survive, it emits endorphins to relieve the pain. The first few times in the water are an enormous

49

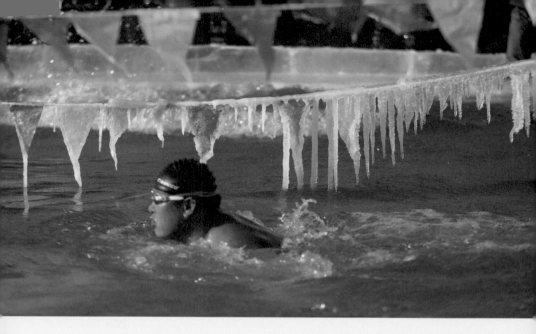

Above: A swimmer competes in a pool carved from thick ice covering the Songhua river during the Harbin Ice Swimming Competition in Heilongjiang province, China.

challenge for both body and mind, but the reward is the euphoric pleasure of endorphins, dopamine and noradrenalin that warm your body when you go home.

Pros and cons

Some people experience overwhelming fatigue when they first begin cold-water swimming. This feeling will fade with increased habituation to the cold water. If you start swimming when the water is at its coldest, the body remembers how challenging it was, both mentally and physically, and for some people this may be enough to dissuade them from doing it again.

For others, beginning in the winter is the perfect model. It all depends on the initial motivation. Many people start in the coldest months to get the biggest thrill and kick from the icy water. They are often tenacious and see the habituation as personal challenge, and the fact that they feel the effects of the cold so intensely may be all it takes for them to keep going. The cold makes it difficult to think about everyday chores, and the icy deep can be a form of resetting the mind from mental overload.

If you choose the winter model and you're hesitating about your second swim, remember that feeling in your body when you got out of the water the first time. Remember the heat that spread throughout your body and the energy that fills you. To start swimming in the winter requires impressive discipline, but the rewards are great.

With the summer model, it can safely be said that there may be a higher success rate for becoming a regular winter swimmer. However, there is longer to wait until the day you get your first real cold shock (which may be Christmas Eve). An exact temperature threshold for the cold-shock response will vary from person to person, but the temperature differentials of body, air and water are probably key. If you are very warm and lower yourself into water that is 15°C (60°F) or even less cold, the temperature difference might cause you to gasp for air. With the winter model, the water is shockingly cold without habituation. You may get the "gift" of the cold water immediately, but the success rate is lower as it is energy-intensive and you're not already in the habit. The summer and winter models have different advantages, but the main thing is that you act on your desire and keep going.

Sea, lake, lido or beach?

The experience is a bit different, depending on whether you jump into the sea from a rock or harbour, head out from the beach or swim in a lake or lido. The salt in seawater makes it warmer compared to the fresh water in lakes. In lakes you are more likely to find slush or ice, which experienced swimmers seek every year. Lakes that are fed by streams from the mountains (for example in Norway, Sweden, Germany and Switzerland) are cold all year round.

Walking into the sea from the beach can feel extra cold because the body is exposed to it only gradually. It is not as pleasant as plunging the body in all at once. A way to overcome this is to wear water shoes, to hurry as far out as you can and immerse your body, including your shoulders. The cold then feels more uniform on the body, and it is easier to control your breathing.

Morning or evening?

You have no doubt seen stunning pictures of sunrises and sunsets that winter swimmers diligently post all over social media. Wow! It's so beautiful and life-affirming, and even more so when you're standing there yourself.

If you are new to winter swimming, however, it can be an advantage to start in the afternoon or evening, because you are more sensitive to the cold in the morning. The core temperature of the body is lowest in the morning (36.5°C/97.7°F) and highest in the evening (37–37.5°C/98.6–99.5°F). Swimming in the afternoon is recommended only for the first few weeks or months, depending on how often you swim, to make the experience as pleasant as possible. But it is just as important to swim when you and your swim buddy can make the time.

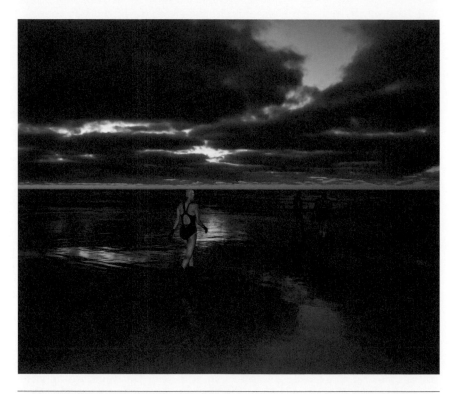

Above: Members of Brighton Swimming Club enjoy a Christmas morning dip. The club is Britain's oldest, founded in 1860.

COLD FACTS:
HOW TO GET INTO THE WATER

- Stay in the habit of swimming after the summer ends and you'll gradually get used to colder water. Or start in the winter months and experience the cold shock more intensely – feel how the body quickly gets used to the cold water.

- Practise before you start swimming by taking cold showers – begin with five seconds and increase up to several minutes.

- You are more sensitive to the cold in the morning. For a beginner, it is better to swim later in the day.

- If you enter the water from a beach, wear swim shoes and wade out to a point where you can be fully immersed.

- Don't worry if to begin with you still feel the chill several hours after your plunge. This is the afterdrop, a normal physiological reaction to cold immersion. It will decrease once you get used to the cold.

- Sign up with a winter swimming club or join an established group.

CHAPTER 4

BAPTISM BY FIRE

"The greatest joy in life is doing
what people say you can't"

WALTER BAGEHOT
Businessman, journalist and economist

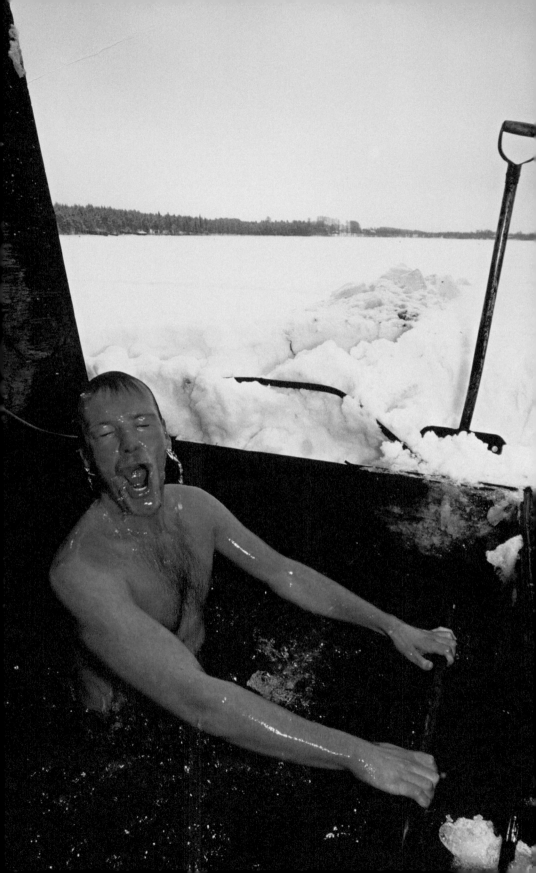

4

So, now you're ready – it's exciting! You need to get used to the cold water, and the first dip is the most difficult one. Choose a day when the conditions are favourable, within reason – without wind and high waves.

On a winter's day in March, I followed two swimmers on a cold-water swim. For one it was his first plunge, and for the other it was something he had tried a few times before. I interviewed them before and after. They were excited and let me watch and record what happens when they got into the water. Their reactions are classic examples of how the body and brain react during the cold-shock response. If you are already a winter swimmer, think back to your first time in the water – do you recognize anything?

9 March 2019, 2 p.m.
INTERVIEW 1
We met on a bench in a small garden outside Svanemøllens Winter Swimming Club. The club is for members only and has a wonderful sauna, but there's a long waiting list to join. We were not members, but we wanted to use the outdoor changing room there and the steps down to the sea. It was a little windy and cold, but the sun was shining. All in all a lovely winter's day, and I could see the new winter swimmer

was excited. We started the interview with the topic at hand – his imminent baptism by fire!

"Hi, let's get started with a little about you, what's your name, your age?"

"I'm André, and I'm twenty-four years old."

"Have you tried winter swimming before?"

"No, never."

"How did you decide that winter swimming was something that you wanted to try?"

"I read an article about this place, it said there was a long waiting list. I thought, if there's a long waiting list there must be something in it. It could be a lot of fun to try!"

"Why do you want to get started now?"

"It's because I read that article – we'll see if it's something for me ... we'll see ..."

"What do you think it's like to get into the cold water?"

"I kind of hope that it's a bit shocking. That you get an out-of-body experience. That the body will react in some way. That there is some adrenalin in the body without it being dangerous."

"Is there anything that you're nervous about in terms of getting into the water? Something you've been thinking about?"

"No, not really, not other than getting ill. Otherwise, I don't think so – these are reasonably controlled conditions."

"Yes. Would you like to become a member of a winter swimming club?"

"We'll see how it goes today, but if I like it, it could be fun also to use the sauna and maybe get to know the community around it."

"So, it's primarily those two things that are interesting – the sauna and the community?"

"We'll have to see how many people there are [on the waiting list]. For example, if I came here with some friends, it might be super fun to do something a little different together. So I think that could be very cool. And to have a place to do it. The fact that it isn't just some random place to go and swim – there's also a place to go and get warm afterwards."

"Would there be anything that would stop you from continuing to winter swim?"

"Not specifically. If anything, it would have to be if it doesn't feel good. And if you had to do it alone. I don't think it'd be that great to have to come out here alone and jump into the cold water and then scurry home again."

We finished the interview and André went into the changing room.

INTERVIEW 2

While André is getting changed, the second winter swimmer sat down on the bench and, like André, he also seemed excited.

"Can you tell me your name and how old you are?"

"My name is Christopher and I'm twenty-three years old."

"Have you ever gone winter swimming before?"

"No . . . well, yes, I tried it before but it's not something I do frequently."

"When did you last do it?"

"Sometime in October, if you can call that winter swimming?"

"You can definitely call it winter swimming. What made you think that you'd want to try it?"

"Because I've just moved close to the water, and one of my friends told me about Svanemøllens Winter Swimming Club – and it just seems fun. And it looks like people have a great time doing it. I once had an old primary school teacher who did it. So it's been stuck in my head since then."

"Why do you want to get started now?"

"Before, I didn't really like the water, but then I did my military service and I got over it a little bit because we went into the water when it was cold. Now I've got used to the fear, and I just think it could be fun to try."

"How do you think it feels to get into the cold water?"

"I imagine it's really cold! [We laugh.] I think it's refreshing and it clears your mind. When you're in, you are just in it – and then you get out, and then you probably can't think about much. My answers afterwards may reflect that. [We laugh.]"

"It'll be interesting! What do you imagine happens in your body?"

"It may be that the cold might be painful somehow, but what happens is probably that you get out and have to use a lot of energy warming yourself up. I can imagine that you feel really tired afterwards."

"Is there anything you're nervous about?"

"Maybe the shock, and maybe the moment just before – standing there and fluttering in the wind – and whether I have the nerve to do it? Once I'm in, it's not going to be hard to get out again!"

"How are you going to get into the water?"

"I'll just jump in. It has to be quick. I'll dive in head first!"

"Head first? That's not usually recommended."

"No? For f**** sake!"

"Would you like to join a winter swimming club?"

"Yes, because it looks so nice with the sauna. When we go out and swim now, we'll have to stand and dry off in the wind, and it'll probably be really cold. And I love going to the sauna. The sauna is a big part of the community. That's where one can seek refuge afterwards. And have fun and bragging rights."

"Is there anything that could stop you from taking this up as a habit?"

"Yeah, if there wasn't a sauna. I don't think I could make myself do it if I had to get up, dry off and cycle home every time."

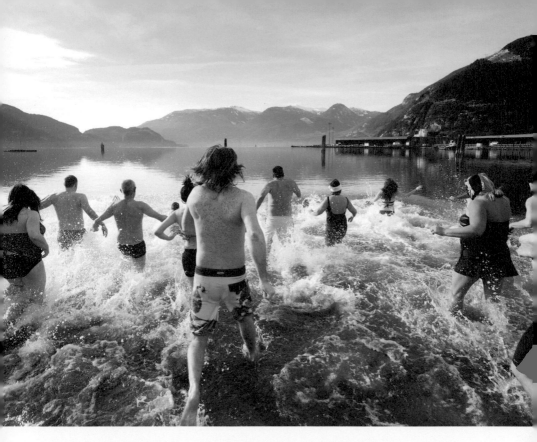

Above: Swimmers enter the water at noon on New Year's Day during the annual Squamish Polar Bear Swim in Howe Sound, near Vancouver, Canada.

We end the interview. Christopher goes to the locker room to change. In a little while they will be in the water!

On the jetty, 2.17 p.m. – André's baptism by fire

We walk onto the jetty. André seems relatively calm; he gets his towel ready on the railing. The stairs down to the water are steep, and in just seven or eight steps his feet will hit the water. We look down at the clear, cold water.

> *"So, André, are you ready to try winter swimming for the first time?"*
> "Yes."
> He walks purposefully down the steps and swims a few strokes.
> "Hu hu huuuuhu!" he pants. After three more strokes, he grabs

the railing and hurriedly climbs up the ladder. At the top of the steps in the wind, André looks miserable; shoulders pulled up to his ears, a stiff smile, and you can hear him gasping for breath.

"How are you feeling right now?"

"I . . . heck . . . not great!" he exclaims, slinging a slightly too small towel around his shoulders.

"What does it feel like?"

"It feels a little like needles on my body," he says, shifting from one leg to the other.

"And how about your head - can you focus?"

"Yes, kind of." André's face looks a little strained, but I dare to ask him anyway:

"Do you feel like doing it again?"

"Not right now, no," André replies, his eyes searching for the changing room.

"Do you need to warm up a little?"

"Yes! . . . No, I'm not going in again, at least not right now!"

"Well done."

André walks towards the building with his towel pulled well up to his ears.

Christopher's swim

We stand on the jetty by the steps. Christopher smiles excitedly.

"Are you ready?"

"Yes," he replies, walking down the steps just as purposefully as André did.

From the water I can hear "Huuu huuu huuuh!" He swims away from the ladder, takes a few strokes and turns towards the ladder again. "F*** - I'm getting OUT!"

"Nice! Can I hand you your towel?"

Someone shouts from the quay, "Well done!"

"Thank you, thank you - I'll just take that," he says, grabbing

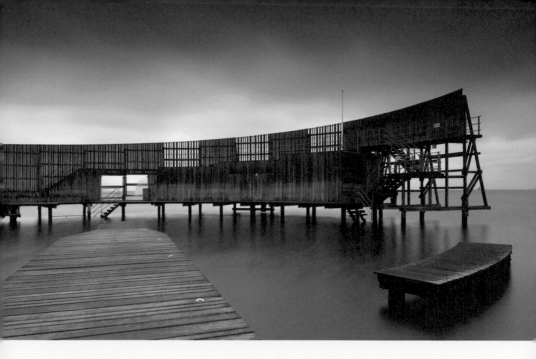

Above: The award-winning Kastrup Sea Bath, Copenhagen, Denmark, offers good swimming with protection against the wind. The circular building is constructed from durable azobé wood and is known as the "Snail" ("*Sneglen*").

the towel I'm holding out. The wind is clearly making him even colder. Christopher wraps the towel around himself, turns and smiles.

"OK, you just got out of the water. How are you feeling right now?"

"Egh – it's actually not that bad right now, I'd say . . . but I can tell by my feet that I'm not going to be able feel them soon." He laughs briefly.

"Would you like to try again?"

"Uh – not right now. No, thanks."

"Is it what you expected?"

"Uh, yeah, kind of, I can't feel that much right now. So, in that way, yes. Thoughts are flying around in my head right now."

"That's how it is when you've just given your body a cold shock."

"Yes, a shock – yes."

"Well done. I'd better let you go now."

"Thank you!" he replies and hurries to the changing room.

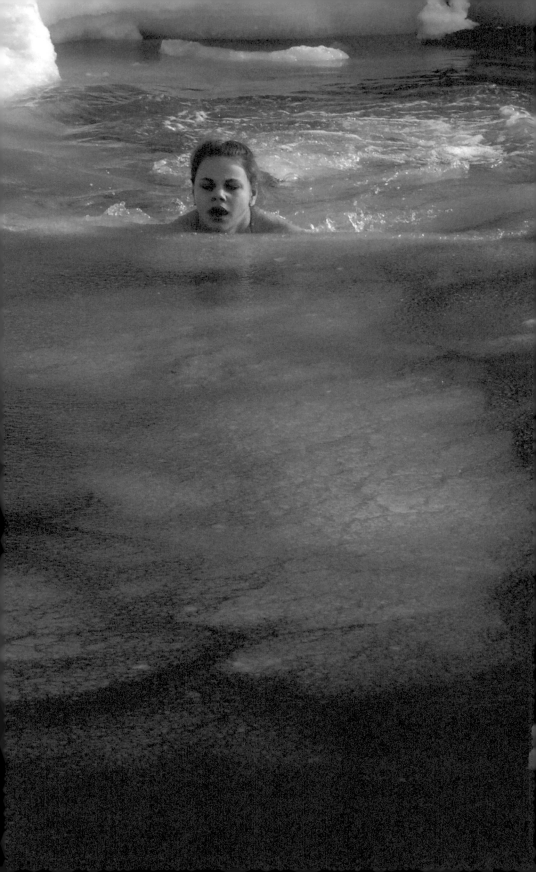

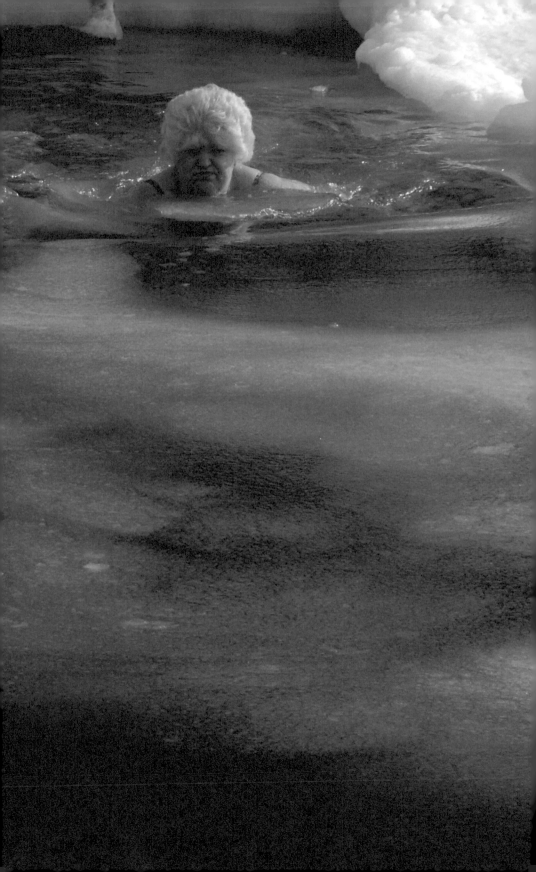

It was clear that André and Christopher got a little addled from the cold. The cold slows the blood flow to the brain, numbs the facial muscles and nerves, and the ability to speak becomes impaired. However, with increasing cold habituation, it becomes easier to control the facial muscles and keep calm. When you get out of the water, the body naturally calls for HEAT, and that instinct in itself shifts your focus away from conversation. But there is also a physiological explanation. Both young men had difficulty describing their feelings and thoughts right after their plunge, which is an effect of the cold-shock response. Adrenalin and noradrenalin trigger the sympathetic nervous system – the flight-or-fight response – and then endorphins, which with the vasoconstriction effect of noradrenalin dull the nerves. The skin becomes numb and simultaneously a slightly euphoric feeling emerges. As demonstrated with the two unhabituated winter swimmers, the cold shock often results in addled, slow speech and a difficulty articulating thoughts and feelings right after cold immersion. It could be described as a brief reset of thoughts and emotions, or a "slow-motion" effect.

The body's reflexes

The first encounter with cold water can be experienced very differently, depending on how you mentally prepare for and cope with the first plunge. Going back a bit in time, I had an experience that was abundantly clear to me. It was the first time I witnessed someone taking their first plunge, and before I became a winter swimmer myself. It was spring and the water was very cold. I hadn't yet started recruiting subjects for our experiments. To see how an initial introduction to the water might be conducted, I met with an experienced winter swimmer along with a brave first-timer. I had just begun my research and thought that a little fieldwork would be enlightening. The beginner went into the water.

Pages 64–65: Participants in a winter swimming competition, Vladivostok, Russia.

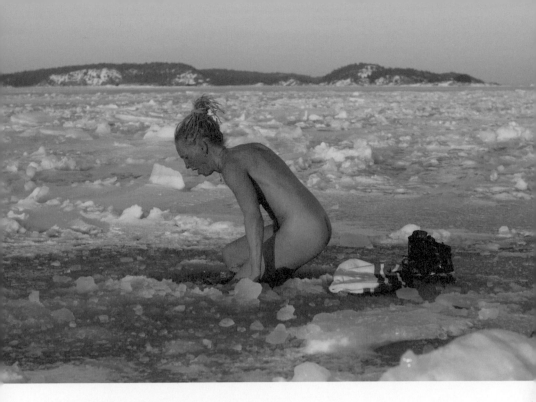

Above: Nudity can be practical.

"AAH [gasping sounds] AAH [gasp] AAAAAAH [gasp] AAAAAH [gasp] AAAARHHHH [gasp]!" he shouted and went on: "AAAAAAH [gasp] AAAAAH [gasp] AAAARHHHH [gasp]!"

I stood on the jetty in a nice warm wool jacket, hat and gloves. The two swimmers were in the ice-cold water, everyone on the beach and the jetty was looking at us. The cold-shock response can be dangerous, especially the first few times, because you gasp instinctively at the shock of cold and there is a risk of choking in water. He shouted and gasped so loudly that I was sure most of this end of Copenhagen could hear it! I myself was completely startled, and immediately felt as though I should save him. "COME OUT NOW!" I called. He didn't hear me and I had to call louder. It must have been comical to watch this action-packed scene. It was clearly a mental challenge for him to feel the cold so intensely. I looked up and saw people walking their dog on the beach stopping to see what torture experiment was going on.

Mental strategies

The cold-shock response comes as a surprise; screams and other sounds are a body's reflex, signalling its shock. Although the whole session probably didn't last for more than fifteen seconds, the screaming felt like it went on for ever. When he got out of the water, he was jubilantly happy and hurried off to the sauna. Meanwhile, I thought about the cold-shock response and came to the conclusion that I had probably interpreted his sounds as panic, when in fact it was his way of dealing with the cold and staying in longer. Impressively, he stayed in the water for longer than most beginners would have done. He was obviously excited, and afterwards he was glad he'd made it through. It was a success. I hope, however, that over time he found new strategies to deal with the cold.

In general, the vast majority of new winter swimmers would not be able to stay in the water long enough for the initial cold-stress response phase to subside. And it isn't advisable either. Mental strategies can be advised for building up habituation but not for the first-time plunge. After two or three times, the body becomes familiar with the cold in a safe way, and you can begin to increase your time spent in the water. It takes between twenty seconds and a minute before the initial calmer phase sets in, where the skin approaches the same temperature as the water and the nerves are numbed by the pain-relieving effect of the endorphins and noradrenalin. It hurts a little less and the water feels less cold. The worst of the stress is over, which makes breathing calmer and more controlled. When you get to this point you've already made great strides in getting acclimatized to the cold.

Opposite: Swimming in an ice hole in the frozen Dnieper river, Dnipro, Ukraine.

Pages 70–71: Determined swimmers at Świnoujście, Poland.

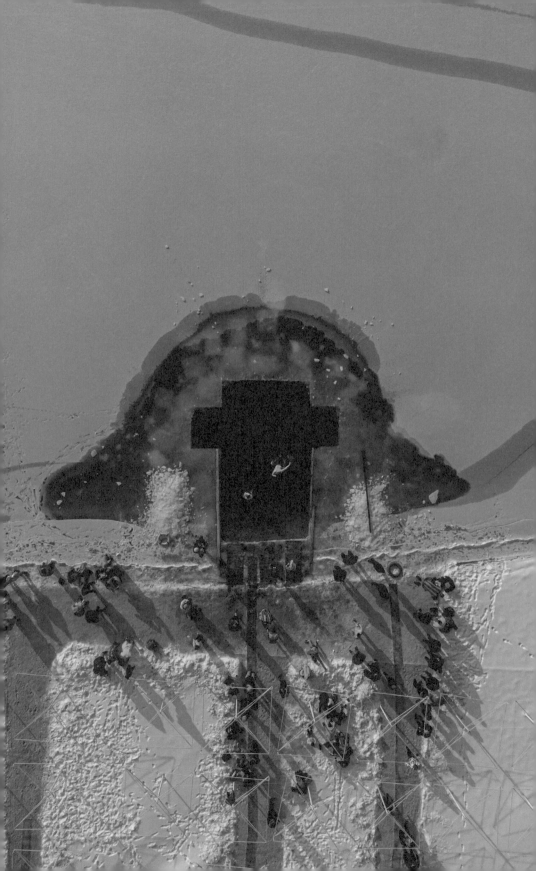

COLD FACTS: *THE FIRST SWIM*

- Never swim alone.

- Warm up your muscles before you go in, with some star jumps or a quick run.

- Keep your robe on all the way to the steps of the jetty. Walk slowly, as the jetty and steps can be slippery.

- Never dive into cold water headfirst.

- Breathe calmly when sitting or swimming in the water – cold water can give you temporary shortness of breath – therefore exhale completely and then go in, breathing deeply and calmly.

- If there are waves, hold on to a rope or railing.

- Go in purposefully until the water covers your shoulders.

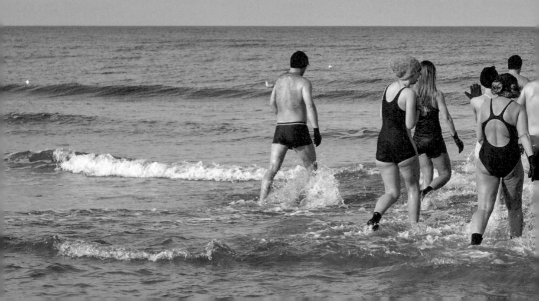

- Take only a short swim of five to ten seconds the first few times.

- Count aloud to occupy your brain in the water. (You can increase your time as you get more and more comfortable with the cold. Most winter swimmers increase by twenty to forty seconds per session.) Then get out of the water and put your bathrobe on. Put your hands in your armpits to warm them up and get over the worst of the cold shock.

- Put on warm clothes and drink plenty of tea or another hot drink.

- If you go directly from the sauna, let your body cool down a bit in the wind before you get into the water – this helps you avoid the worst of the cold shock.

- Under no circumstances go into the water if you feel ill or are under the influence of alcohol.

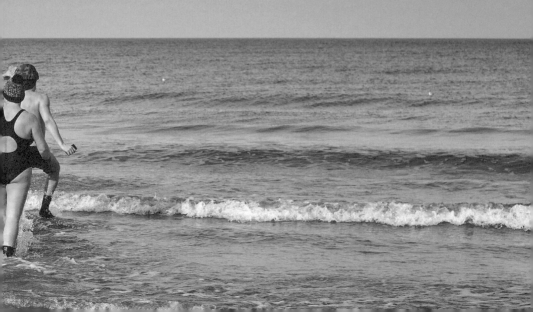

CHAPTER 5

THE COLD-SHOCK RESPONSE

"You cannot swim for new horizons until you have
the courage to lose sight of the shore"
WILLIAM FAULKNER
Writer and Nobel laureate

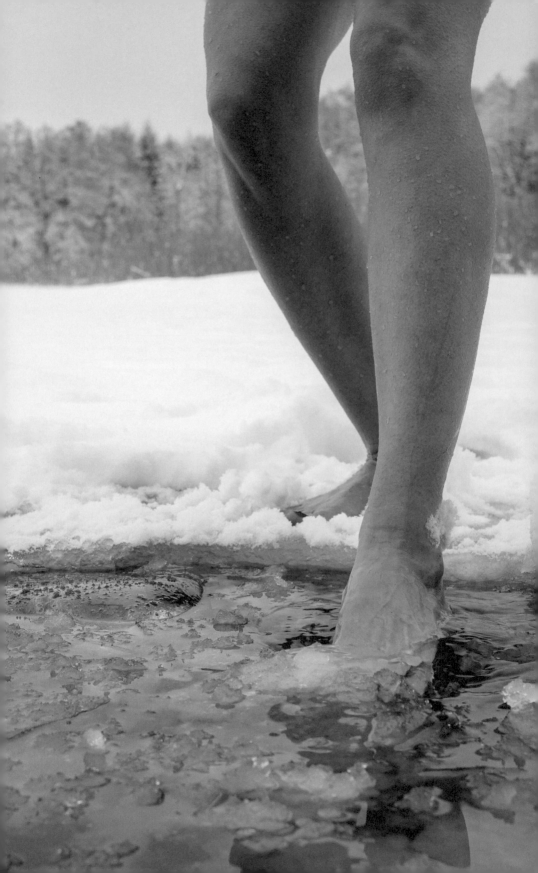

5

The blood rushes through your veins and you gasp audibly for breath. The cold water feels like needles on your skin. This feeling lasts for a minimum of twenty seconds, if you have practised winter swimming, after which you gradually feel calmer and your breathing settles. Due to the cold-shock response, your skin grows numb, and when you get out of the water, peripheral veins will dilate and a feeling of heat starts flowing through your body. This could be a description of the physiological feeling of a winter swim.

What happens in your body?

When winter swimming, the two factors affecting the body are the cold and the hydrostatic pressure of water. As mentioned previously, the cardiovascular response experienced by unhabituated winter swimmers on initial immersion in cold water is known as the "cold-shock response". It is defined as a reflex response driven by the sympathetic system due to the activation of peripheral cold receptors, and it manifests itself as an inspiratory gasp followed by hyperventilation, tachycardia (increased heart rate) and hypertension. The decrease in skin temperature activates cold receptors. The physiological explanation is that cold receptors in the skin signal to the hypothalamic temperature centre in the brain. In other words, they send a message saying "THIS IS SUPER COLD!!", and the brain responds by activating the sympathetic nervous system. The sympathetic activation promotes cutaneous vasoconstriction, tachycardia, brown adipose tissue thermogenesis and neurons that cause shivering in the skeletal muscle to generate heat. This escalation prevents the body from becoming hypothermic.

The cold-shock response happens when cold water touches your skin, either during complete immersion or during cold showers, triggering an increase in heart rate and blood pressure. At the same time the parasympathetic system is activated due to the "diving response" associated with cold-water immersion, which, contrary to the sympathetic nervous system, lowers heart rate and blood pressure. Could it be that there is a physiological conflict in the system during cold-water immersion? Yes, this could well be the case and explains what winter swimmers feel before and after the initial cold shock: hyperventilation, which gradually turns to normal breathing and feeling calm.

What happens is that the hydrostatic pressure caused by cold-water immersion stimulates baroreceptors (both arterial and cardiopulmonary), resulting in an inhibition of the sympathetic nervous system and an increase in vagal tone. Vagal tone is the activity of the vagus nerve (the tenth cranial nerve and a fundamental component of the parasympathetic branch of the autonomic nervous system) and gets its name from the fact that it involves an interplay between the nerve and your blood vessels. Activation of the vagal nerve is not within our conscious control, and is largely responsible for the regulation of several internal body functions at rest, including heart-rate

Opposite: Epiphany ice-hole swimming at Lake Shartash, Yekaterinburg, Russia.

Page 74: Go slowly, but steadily, into the water and accept the fact that it's cold.

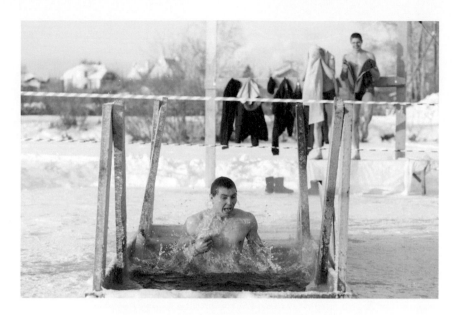

reduction, vasodilation/constriction of vessels, lungs, digestive tract, liver and immune system regulation as well as inflammation. Cold-water immersion therefore results in bradycardia (lowered heart rate) and a decrease in total peripheral resistance, because it inhibits the constriction of the vessels caused by the sympathetic nervous system.

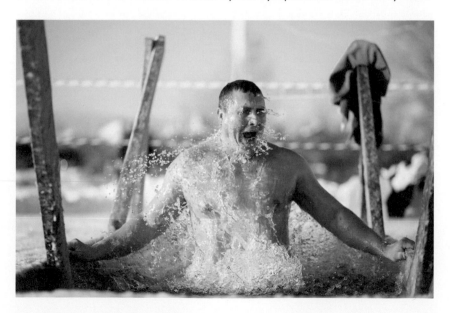

According to a couple of older physiology studies from 1995 and 2000, these two opposing responses can occur at the same time when the body is immersed in cold water. A summary of the published data in studies of unhabituated individuals revealed almost no change in blood pressure and heart rate as a result of the conflicting systems during cold-water immersion after the initial shock (about thirty seconds to one minute).

As previously mentioned, the cold-shock response consists of inspiratory gasps, hyperventilation and tachycardia in the first two to three minutes of immersion if you are an unhabituated winter swimmer. Gradually, with habituation, the cold-shock response time will decrease. Let me explain how the cold-shock response works in practice: when you enter the water, everything kicks in, and involuntarily you begin to gasp for air and to hyperventilate, especially if you're not used to swimming in the cold. The brain immediately perceives the icy water as dangerous. The shock triggers the stress response in which the body focuses on surviving and protecting its most vital organs. Peripheral blood vessels in fingers, toes, arms, legs and skin contract quickly. The blood flows towards the core to maintain heat, oxygen and functions in the vital organs. The heart rate drops due to the diving response and the heart no longer needs to pump blood all the way to the small blood vessels in the extremities, which lowers the blood pressure. Studies in the acute cardiovascular response of cold-water immersion show a small increase in blood pressure immediately before unhabituated winter swimmers go into the water. This is probably due to excitement and nervousness over the impending cold rush.

What happens in your brain

The cold shock also causes blood flow to the brain to drop by as much as 30 per cent. In a study from 2007, thirteen male unacclimatized volunteers were lowered into a 0°C (32°F) immersion tank for exactly half a minute. Within seconds after immersion, their heart rate increased on average from 74 to 107 beats per minute, and their respiratory rate from 16 to 38 breaths per minute, and two subjects showed signs of imminent syncope (drowsiness, blurred vision, loss of responsiveness). Decreased blood flow and increased respiratory rate can cause dizziness with an associated risk of loss of consciousness, falling and ensuing trauma to the head. So, there's good reason to be careful and to take it slowly at the beginning! You don't have to put your head under water, as this will increase the cold-shock response, and the risk of syncope and drowning. It is important to note that an inexperienced winter swimmer is unlikely to stay in ice-cold water for thirty seconds, as in the above-mentioned experiment. Instead, the advice is to take a few seconds' dip at a time, and to build up cold adaptation slowly. If you feel dizziness and tingling in your eyes, it is important that you get out of the water and bend your head down to heart level until you feel the blood supply to the brain again.

It has long been known that exposure to cold of the kind that we experience during winter swimming reduces the cognitive functions of the brain, and that general brain activity is reduced by temperature drops. But even if your speech gets a little slurred, it doesn't mean that you can't think logically the moment you are in the water; it's simply that the cold shock takes your focus away from anything other than the cold. Cold shock is something of a "slow-motion button" for your brain.

A cascade of hormones and neural activation

While you're in the water, your body works to survive the extreme threat of the cold; it begins to produce heat by increasing your metabolism to keep your blood warm and to keep you awake. The question is whether the physiological changes can have health-promoting effects in addition to helping the body get used to the cold water. There are some indications to suggest that this is the case. The stress response consists mainly of three hormones: adrenalin, noradrenalin and cortisol. As a reaction to this cascade of hormones, the secretion of several other hormones will follow – endorphins, dopamine and serotonin – along with neural signalling in the brain. This gives you a feeling of happiness and mental balance.

The cold water triggers cold shock immediately, releasing hormones in the body and activating neurotransmitters in the brain to protect you from the dangers of the cold. The hormones and neurons in the central nervous system increase at the same time, resulting in several different healthy outcomes. But are the hormones or neural signalling the main driver for the effects of the cold water?

A study from 2000 measured hormonal release in both warm (32°C and 20°C/90°F and 68°F) and cold water (14°C/57°F). The scientists found that physiological changes brought about by water immersion are mediated by humoral control mechanisms (meaning the hormones that are released into the blood when the body is immersed in water), while responses induced by the cold are mainly due to increased activity of the sympathetic nervous system and neurotransmitters. So, during winter swimming, the cold temperature causes mainly neural activation and is probably the main driver of the different effects: enhanced mood and mental balance. It makes sense that the body, like a motorway, sends messages to the brain and back to the skin to contract in order to protect the vital organs from hypothermia and to survive. Hormones increase too, however the responses are probably too slow to save us in the initial moments. An example is adrenalin, which is generally rapidly increased as a neurotransmitter on cold immersion, but not when measured as a hormone in the blood. Neural activation is rapid in the cold – like lightning – whereas hormones such as adrenalin and noradrenalin are produced in the adrenal glands. This process is slower. So in terms of survival during cold immersion, neural activation is what saves us from becoming hypothermic. It is difficult to measure neurotransmitters in the human brain, however, and we need further studies to gain insight into neural responses during cold-water immersion.

GETTING INTO COLD WATER

Parasympathetic nervous system
Is activated and stabilizes serotonin. Vagal tone stimulated.

Brain
30% less blood flow to the brain prompts reduction of cognitive functions. Noradrenalin and serotonin are increased in the brain with positive effects on mood.

Lungs
Gasping reflex triggered; hyperventilation.

Heart
Greater blood flow to heart and internal organs, resulting in lower heart rate and stroke volume.

Panic?
No: the cold shock subsides. Endorphins numb pain in the skin and the skin approaches water temperature. Breathing and pulse become calmer.

Peripheral blood vessels
Contract in the skin, hands and toes.

Brown fat
Is activated, using sugar and fat from the bloodstream as fuel to keep warm.

Skin
Beta receptors in the skin engage the parasympathetic nervous system.

Muscle tremors?
When the brown fat can no longer maintain body temperature, muscle tremors occur.

The sympathetic nervous system
Adrenalin, noradrenalin and cortisol increase as part of the fight-or-flight response. Dopamine and endorphins increase.

The immune system
Boosted by an increase of white blood cells, monocytes and a larger antioxidant system.

Adrenalin

First, the body responds to the external stress (ice-cold water) with neural activation and the secretion of adrenalin. Adrenalin is a combat hormone which heightens your awareness and awakens your fight-or-flight response. It acts as a neurotransmitter in the central nervous system and is a hormone produced in the adrenal medulla – a small organ that lies above the kidneys. Adrenalin binds to cells and is responsible for various physiological effects. For example, when we get into ice-cold water, adrenalin acts on the surface of the liver and muscle cells, signalling to the cells to release glucose into the bloodstream from their large glycogen stores. That way, the muscles have access to glucose to generate more energy to respond to the potentially life-threatening situation of being in cold water. The blood vessels in the muscles and heart dilate as they narrow in the skin, increasing blood flow and the availability of glucose for the inner organs and muscles. At the same time, the production of insulin decreases to maintain high glucose levels in the blood – rapid energy for the fight-or-flight challenge you have put yourself up to!

Endorphins

Due to the increase in catecholamines (noradrenalin, adrenalin and cortisol), cold-water swimming could be a treatment for depression as it activates the sympathetic nervous system and increases the concentration of noradrenalin and beta-endorphin. If cold showers or winter swimming are not your thing, it is very likely that standard exercise, such as a run, would have the same effect. It is believed that endorphins as neurotransmitters are released at the same time as adrenalin in the brain. It is the body's own drug that cheers you up and makes you happy. Endorphins are primarily analgesic, and they are needed because the cold causes your body intense pain. Endorphins are also increased, for example, when you work out, achieve success, fall in love, have sex or laugh. Synthetic endorphins can also be found, for example, in chocolate. Endorphins are more potent than morphine

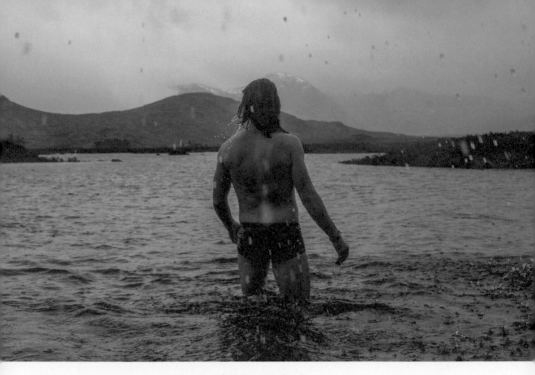

Above: Braving the elements, Isle of Skye, Scotland.

and they are addictive. Winter swimming is therefore an activity that can make you both happy and addicted, and so it is an easy habit to maintain.

Noradrenalin

Noradrenalin is often secreted alongside adrenalin – the two hormones have almost the same effects in the body – and it's also a hormone that is produced in stressful situations. It acts both as a hormone and as a neurotransmitter in the brain. The hormonal noradrenalin is secreted from the adrenal gland, like adrenalin, and acts as a kind of combat hormone which, together with adrenalin, usually raises heart rate and blood pressure when we experience danger. It also helps to keep us awake and alert. In addition, noradrenalin is the hormone and neural signal that most effectively activates the brown fat to increase heat and metabolism during cold exposure – much more about this in Chapter 7 (Brown Fat). So, noradrenalin originates from two different areas, the adrenal medulla (80 per cent adrenalin, 20 per cent noradrenalin) and the sympathetic activation of nerves and release of neurotransmitters.

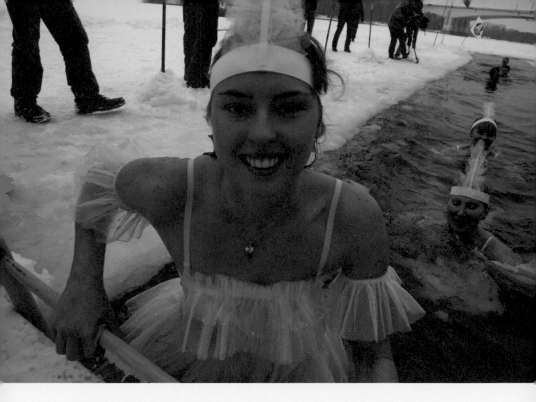

Above: Members of the Capital Walruses winter swimming club participate in ice-hole swimming competitions in Moscow, Russia.

Under normal circumstances only very small amounts of noradrenalin from the sympathetic nerve endings reach circulation as the majority is either recaptured (75 per cent) or degraded locally (25 per cent). However, during high sympathetic activity, as with winter swimming, the released noradrenalin from the sympathetic nerves increases to a high level and reaches circulation, like a spillover. This can cause a large increase of noradrenalin in the blood.

I investigated the literature to examine how much adrenalin and noradrenalin we can measure in the blood upon cold-water immersion. Surprisingly, all the studies seem to agree that no changes in adrenalin occurred. However, studies measuring noradrenalin in the blood within three minutes of cold-water immersion agree that an increase occurs. One study also reported a repeated increase in noradrenalin in experienced winter swimmers undertaking brief swims of less than three minutes over three months of winter swimming. Part of the body's cold-shock response is a stress response that manifests as an up to four-fold increase in noradrenalin. One study measured noradrenalin continuously before, during and after cold-water immersion, and recorded an immediate increase in noradrenalin within two minutes of immersion, followed by a continuous increase in concentration throughout the immersion. From the rapid increase it may be assumed that noradrenalin release is connected to changes in skin temperature rather than in core temperature. This supports the idea – and indeed my advice – that the health benefits of cold-water immersion do not depend on a drop in the core temperature, and so long winter swims or dips of fifteen minutes or more are not necessary. In some cases this will increase the risk of hypothermia and other cold-induced conditions described in later chapters.

Cortisol

The thyroid-stimulating hormone that controls metabolism, cortisol, is the third stress or combat hormone, and it is also released from the adrenal glands in stressful situations or during fasting, when the body needs energy. Cortisol contributes to an increase in blood sugar and also works by breaking down the body's energy stores. In this way, energy is generated for demanding situations. Studies have shown that winter swimmers have higher levels of cortisol during cold-water immersion and after a swimming season. However, cortisol levels when the body is at rest may be lower upon habituation. That's fortunate, because it turns out that cortisol has a strong calming effect on inflammatory conditions in the body, for example in arthritis or atherosclerosis (thickening or hardening of the arteries). It works by inhibiting the immune system, which is responsible for inflammation. Cortisol therefore plays a role in the reduction of inflammation in the blood vessels that we often see in winter swimmers. All in all, the stress response appears to increase metabolism, burning sugar and fat, which is a good start to keeping your body awake and warm. Other hormones that increase are dopamine and serotonin.

Dopamine

Dopamine is a hormone and neurotransmitter that acts as part of the brain's reward system. It is not measured directly in the human brain, but studies on rodents suggest increased neural dopamine release due to the cold-shock response. An increase in dopamine produces a feeling of happiness and contentment. It is therefore extremely addictive and will help you maintain the good habit of jumping into cold water again and again! Studies exploring the long-term effects of cold stress could give us more insight into the effect of habituation to cold.

Dopamine is one of the signal substances that is crucial to our positively motivated actions, the ones we associate with joy and well-being. You can get a dopamine kick in many different situations, such as when you succeed at something, or take certain kinds of drugs, or are in a pleasurable situation. And the signal substance is amplified by the repetition of the pleasurable situation. It is likely that dopamine is the explanation for your increased dedication to go winter swimming, when your brain enjoys the thought of taking a cold dip. At this point you have become a winter swimmer for sure!

Unfortunately, some people develop an imbalance in dopamine levels, where the brain does not produce enough of it; this can lead to depression, addiction, schizophrenia and other mental disorders. In normal conditions, the brain activates its own neurotransmitters when we feel happy and rewarded. When a little dopamine is released in the brain, we feel a diffused well-being. The release of large amounts of dopamine will cause happiness, and extreme amounts will induce a feeling of great joy. This is likely the explanation for the joyful mood winter swimmers describe after taking a plunge. The cold-shock response can trigger a dopamine kick, and could be a natural prevention of depression.

As mentioned earlier, cold-water immersion at 14°C (57°F) increases plasma dopamine levels by 250 per cent. Furthermore, the reheating process (e.g. the sauna) has also shown to increase dopamine to a level that gives a feeling of well-being afterwards.

Serotonin

Like dopamine, serotonin is part of the brain's reward system and is secreted during cold-water immersion. It is most closely associated with mental balance, happiness, relaxation and good sleep, and studies have found that low serotonin signalling in the brain is associated with depression. Serotonin also plays an important role in regulating appetite and memory, and much more. As explained in Chapter 2 (Why Swim in the Winter?), the cold activates the parasympathetic nervous system responsible for rest and repair of the body's cells, and the sympathetic nervous system makes us alert and strong. The cooperation of the two systems – like yin and yang – is necessary to maintain balance in body and mind. Therefore, along with the effects of the hormones and catecholamines from the cold shock itself, serotonin is essential to keep us happy, calm and mentally balanced.

It is possible that cold water has no direct effect on baseline serotonin levels. The part of the brain where serotonin works is probably related to the warming effect in itself. It makes sense, therefore, to raise serotonin levels before and after winter swimming. How? A natural way to do this is by exposing yourself to sunlight – exposure you'll get

Winter swimming produces a joyful intoxication in the body that lasts well after one has come out of the water. Does this make you want to try winter swimming?

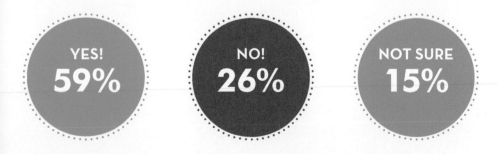

YES! 59%   NO! 26%   NOT SURE 15%

Results of a survey by the author of non-winter swimmers.

anyway when you take a winter swim. There are studies suggesting that too little sunlight contributes to seasonal depression, and that people who are already depressed risk becoming even more depressed if they get too little light. Other ways to increase natural serotonin levels are through exercise, including breathing exercises and massage, and even by remembering to think "happy thoughts". Consciously thinking happy thoughts will activate the parasympathetic nervous system, lower stress and slow breathing. The connection between emotion and temperature has been known for a long time, and it seems there is good reason to take this enforced "happiness thinking" seriously when you get into cold water – it might enhance it even more. In the end, you won't even have to force it. Studies suggest that a positive mindset and a focus on positive memories can make you feel physically warmer and more balanced mentally.

Opposite: Taking the plunge in Vilnius, Lithuania. On this sunny winter day in 2012, the air temperature was -20°C (-4°F).

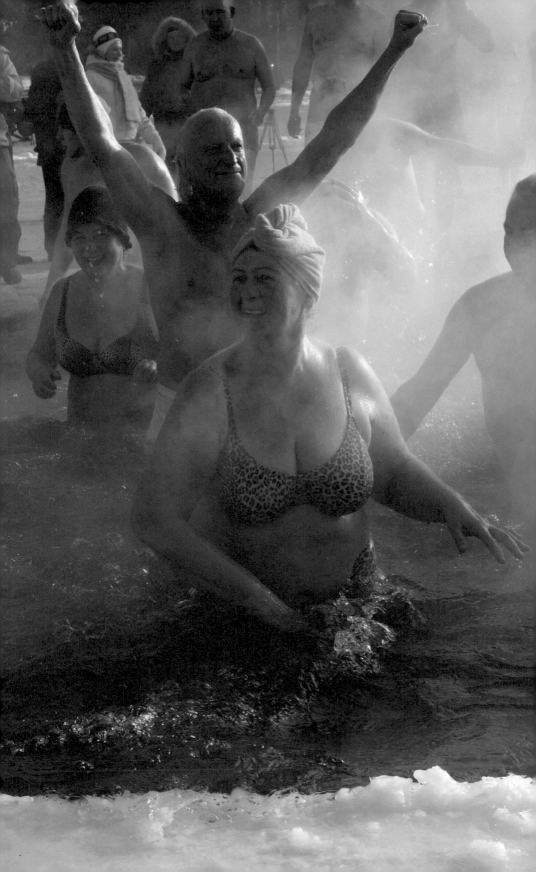

CHAPTER 6

COLD ACCLIMATIZATION

"Excellence is an art won by
training and habituation"

ARISTOTLE
Philosopher and scientist

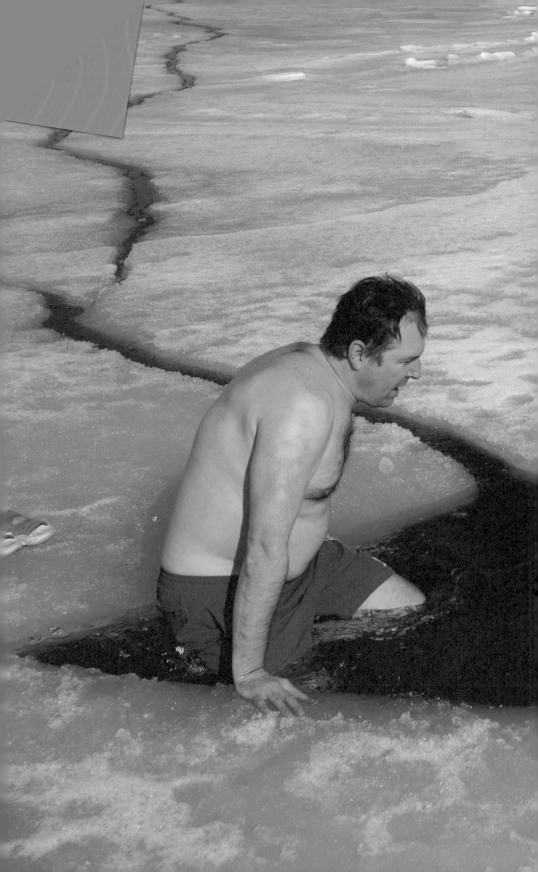

6

The cold shock is overwhelming, but with practice it is possible to build up physiological adaptations to stay in the water longer. At the beginning it's all about discipline and training, and you don't need to stay in the water for very long. Go on a regular basis, but only stay in for as long as feels right, and be sure you understand the signs of hypothermia. Your body will take care of the rest! It's easy – but what actually happens in your body is quite complex.

The balance between metabolic heat production and heat loss is what the body tries to improve for your future cold immersions, and there are three main mechanisms that affect this: habituation, metabolic acclimatization and insulation. Let me briefly explain what we currently know about these three mechanisms.

Habituation

When physiological responses to cold become less pronounced, habituation develops. You can experience this as so-called blunted shivering (less vigorous shivering in skeletal muscles), blunted cutaneous vasoconstrictor response, or both, as compared to the unacclimatized state. Habituation becomes evident as metabolic heat production increases due to shivering, and skin temperature and peripheral heat loss decrease due to vasoconstriction of peripheral blood vessels. It is found that habituation can occur even if parts of the body, such as hands, are exposed to cold. For example, studies in fishermen working with one hand in cold water for many hours have shown that they maintain higher hand and finger temperatures and lower systemic blood pressure than control subjects. But what happens if we dip more than a hand into cold water and do this again and again?

Metabolic acclimatization

Winter swimming is of course much more than dipping a hand into cold water – it's full-body cold-water exposure. There are studies suggesting that repeated exposure to cold can lead to a more pronounced thermogenic response. It is controlled by two mechanisms, which together improve the body's capacity to produce and retain heat, which in turn is crucial to your ability to stay in the water and warm up again after your swim. These mechanisms are responsible for:

- **Improved heat regulation, which is probably due to activation of the brown fat and hormones circulating in the body.**

- **Heat production by muscle shivering.**

Let me elaborate on the two mechanisms. Imagine an early morning on a cold winter's day. You're standing on a jetty, about to go into the water. You take off your bathrobe and hang it on the railing. Now you go down the steps, but you're not nervous, you've done this before. You

---

Page 92: Winter swimming in the frozen Black Sea – a vanishingly rare phenomenon – at Odessa, Ukraine.

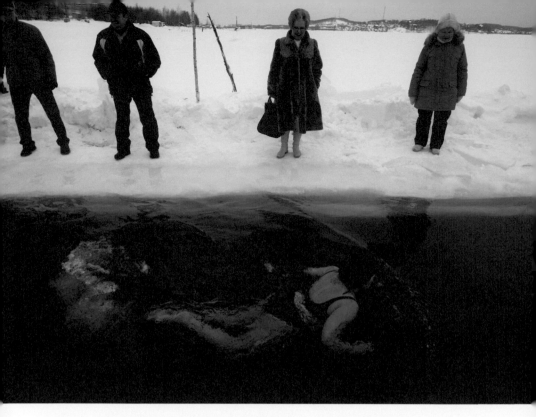

Above: A competitor in a winter swimming tournament at the Verkh-Neyvinsky Pond near Novouralsk, Ural Mountains, Russia.

know you can be in the water longer, compared to when you started winter swimming almost three months ago. So what's happened since then to make it easier?

You get into the water and take a few strokes. Immediately, your metabolism increases and heat production begins. In fact it already started when you undressed in the cold wind. The cold water stimulates a whole range of compensating mechanisms that work to maintain your body temperature. Adrenalin is not the only catecholamine responsible for the fast action of your fight-or-flight response; noradrenalin is too. Noradrenalin increases up to four times above normal levels, as explained in Chapter 5 (The Cold-Shock Response). It results in a warming of the body due to an acute increase in hormones such as cortisol and vasopressin, which regulate blood pressure. This results in an increased metabolism, which in turn increases heat production. The fast increase in metabolism is thought to be mainly due to a relatively unknown but very important organ, brown fat.

Brown fat produces heat as soon as you get into the water and feel the cold – in fact, it is activated as soon as your skin gets cold on single body parts such as hands, feet and face. Noradrenalin activates brown fat, and is the body's most important activator – that's why it's immediately stimulated via your central nervous system when you're in cold water.

Non-shivering thermogenesis

With the help of noradrenalin, the body tries to keep the dangerous cold at bay. It's part of the same thing, namely a mechanism known in research as non-shivering thermogenesis, which really just means: "The heat production that occurs in the body when it is extremely cold, but not yet so cold that the muscles shiver." With this you have kick-started your entire metabolism, that is, your energy burning, which continues long after you have finished your dip, and which is where you get the health benefits of this crazy pastime.

Muscle shivering

It's now been somewhere between seconds and minutes and you're still swimming around in the water. You're in control of your breathing, and you concentrate on staying in the water a little longer. It's going really well so far. But let's assume you keep swimming. This is when it starts to get difficult, as the non-shaking thermogenesis is, at some point, no longer enough to keep your body warm. Your body temperature drops so much that your second heat-producing mechanism now complements the first: heat production by means of muscle shivering.

Muscle shivering produces heat as soon as the muscles start to tremble. Scientific papers appear inconclusive as to the exact point at which the two systems complement each other. The shivering increases gradually with the cold, and probably already starts when you hit the water, as muscles account for the majority of heat production in the body. If you do not possess any brown fat for non-shivering

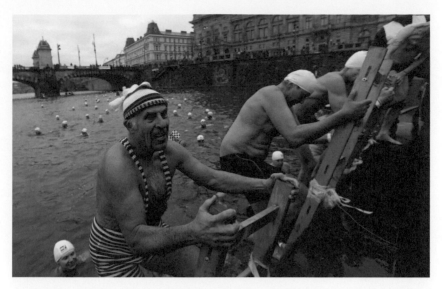

Above: The annual Christmas winter swimming competition in the Vltava, Prague, Czech Republic.

thermogenesis, the muscles will probably start shivering even earlier. If both mechanisms are activated you can stay a little longer in the water without becoming hypothermic. However, the muscles tire due to the hard work, which results in a decrease in muscle coordination, which in turn reduces your ability to swim and perform. Everyone has probably been so cold that they shiver and seen how little control you suddenly have of your hands, feet and speech. Instinctively, you won't want to stay in the water when you start shivering – you have to get out and get warm. Shivering is the first sign of hypothermia, and of a body that's having difficulty keeping its heat production going. At this point you climb up the steps and, shivering, put on your bathrobe and seek heat indoors.

Brain and core

The body's gradual habituation to cold is due to changes in the temperature-regulating centre of the brain, which becomes less sensitive to changes in skin temperature and therefore responds more slowly. On the other hand, your core reacts to a greater degree and for a longer time if its temperature changes. Preferably this wouldn't happen too often or too much, because all your vital organs are located there. The first heat-producing mechanism, non-shivering thermogenesis, is therefore an important mechanism for experienced winter swimmers. Some experienced swimmers can be in the first phase of thermogenesis for many minutes before muscle shivering visibly starts.

Much of the heat is produced from brown fat, and a promising hypothesis is that the more you swim in winter, the more the brown fat is activated, and the longer it is likely to be able to produce heat for you to be able stay in cold water. In untrained winter swimmers, the first heat-producing mechanism without muscle shivering lasts only a short time. Some will get the shivers almost immediately, while others may last a few minutes or more before visible shivering occurs.

To gain more insight into the long-term effects of winter swimming on heart rate and blood pressure as a sign of cardiovascular adaptation, I found studies in which scientists have measured blood pressure before and after a winter swimming season. They show that blood pressure decreases or remains virtually unchanged in habituated winter swimmers.

Blood flow to the skin and insulation

A third, rarely seen, but very important mechanism that can improve through exposure to cold water is the reduction of blood flow to the skin by an increased vasoconstriction response. It acts as a kind of insulation, and with acclimatization, thermal conductance at the skin is lower during cold exposure as compared to that of people in an unacclimatized state. Cold exposure also elicits a more rapid and more pronounced cutaneous vasoconstrictor response with acclimatization. As a result, the vasoconstriction is faster and greater, which leads to a rapid decline in skin temperature during cold exposure. This decline is greater in those who are acclimatized than in those who are not.

Acclimatization to cold water can be helped by:

- Having a layer of white fat on the limbs and torso without being overweight.

- Being able to stay calm in cold water.

- Having the ability to withstand muscle tremors.

- The body's ability to increase its metabolism – the amount of brown fat.

In acclimatized people it works as a way of shutting out the cold, a big shield or a form of insulation. If you ever wonder how cold-water swimmers stay so long in the water and seem fine, this is the reason – a shield consisting of veins contracting and shutting down blood flow to the skin. During vasoconstriction the small blood vessels in the skin contract, which leads to greater blood volume going to the internal organs and a lower pulse with less output from the heart. It is commonly believed that cold water causes the blood to flow faster in the skin and the heart rate to rise. In fact the heart rate drops, as mentioned earlier, during cold-water immersion.

Studies suggest that an extreme form of cold exposure is necessary to build up an insulative mechanism. Scientists took Japanese pearl divers – the Ama women divers – as an example and compared them to non-divers of the same community. They immersed both into cold water and found that the temperature of the Ama divers' skin dropped dramatically compared to the non-divers, which meant that the Ama divers had greater skin tissue insulation. But since Ama divers began to wear wetsuits in the 1970s, this form of insulative acclimatization was no longer evident. It is the physiological adaptation of the three mechanisms that makes winter swimmers more tolerant of cold water.

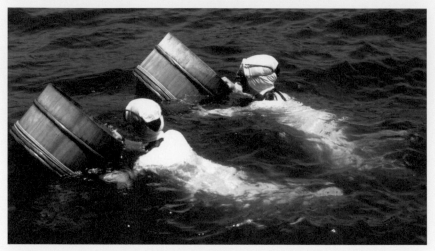

Above: Traditional Japanese Ama pearl divers.

Accepting the cold

It's a cold winter's day, and you tense your body and shiver as you wait at the bus stop. Your shoulders sit right up under your ears. It's tiring. Maybe you have tried to just let go and relax in such a situation. Boom – you lower your shoulders and you stop shivering. Was it just the thought of the cold that made you shiver? Partly. Winter swimmers often talk about learning to accept the cold, to stay calm and avoid panic. It's no surprise that the water is cold when you go for a winter swim, but you're still shocked when you dip your toes in. Can it really be SO cold? Even adapted winter swimmers get surprised by the cold. The cold sensation is never the same, and this makes it exciting to keep going.

As explained earlier in this chapter, we know that getting used to colder temperatures with repeated winter swimming relies on specialized mechanisms in the body. But can it be influenced – pushed, moved, motivated – so that you can swim more, or swim even longer? The answer is yes! The way to do so is to use the mind's acceptance of the cold – and breathing control. In tandem with a build-up of physiological cold resistance, this will help the body relax.

Relax your shoulders

We arrived at the jetty, a female subject from my project and I. We just stood there, enjoying the beautiful morning sun, and we were lucky as the wind wasn't strong that day. In the water was another winter swimmer. We stood chatting about this and that and looking at the water. We both remarked that the man had been swimming in the water for a long time now, we weren't sure exactly but it felt unusually long and he was in no rush to get into the sauna. Before long it was my subject's turn – her baptism by fire! She took a deep breath and went into the changing room.

"Was there something about you guys doing a study?" the man asked on his way up the steps. I replied that we were, and that it was about winter swimming and brown fat. I kept it short so he'd be able to dash away into the sauna. But he still seemed to be in no hurry.

"Exciting!" he said. "How many subjects will there be, and what are you researching?" Impressive, I thought. Very impressive; he stands there in the October cold with only a towel around his waist. Isn't he freezing? When I've been in the water, I move as if pulled by a magnet towards the sauna, but he clearly knows something about accepting the cold. "How can you swim for so long – do you do anything to help you tolerate the cold?" I dared to ask. "At first my brain tried to avoid the cold," he said, "but that didn't work because the cold was there! And it's hard to ignore. Then I tried to accept the cold and everything that was happening in my body. The moment I stopped resisting, my focus on feeling the icy pain on my skin disappeared."

To increase your tolerance of the cold, you can:

- Relax with breathing exercises. Breath in through your nose and out of your mouth.

- Ignore your inner resistance to the cold.

It sounded convincing, but I hadn't asked what he meant by "resisting". It's some years ago now, and since then I have learned that the resistance is one's own mindset – one's expectation that the cold is going to be uncomfortable – "Ugh", we think, and we hunch our shoulders up to our ears, but what we should really do is relax the tension and let them drop. One of the benefits of getting used to the cold and achieving more self-control is that winter swimmers build up cold resistance and don't freeze nearly as much when they're out in cold weather. They're also likely to get the health benefits of the cold-shock response, as long as they don't get hypothermic. This can be an advantage if you work in environments with very low temperatures or live in cold countries – in Russia, for example, winter swimming is used as a means to prepare your body for exposure to the cold.

In the beginning, it's all about patience and slowly getting used to the cold. After you've been in the water about three times, it's already a lot easier to control your breathing, and you've established a good basis for swimming longer.

Performance, fat stores and muscle

Your winter swimming performance also depends on your fat and muscle stores. The body's distribution of fat, muscle mass and general physical shape is of great importance. You build muscle and reduce the amount of white fat through physical exercise. This is easier said than done, but you should see it as a process – you start winter swimming, and you might want to improve. My advice would be get in good shape and achieve a better ratio between fat and muscle – over time you will be able to stay in the water for longer, as muscles produce heat.

Winter swimming, like other sports or physical activities that can be practised at different levels, depends on how much interest, time and energy you want to put into it. If you want to learn to swim in cold water, it's a good idea to build up muscle mass. When we get cold, our sympathetic nervous system is activated and our muscles begin to shiver to produce heat. Muscle cells rapidly absorb oxygen and sugar

If you have a high body fat percentage and start dieting and training alongside winter swimming, your body will show signs of improved health, such as:

- Greater physical and mental energy.

- Greater sense of well-being. This due to the increased endorphins and dopamine hormones produced during the cold-shock response and exercise. The high number of cytokines present in overweight people counteracts the effect of endorphins, dopamine and serotonin.

- Less shortness of breath when climbing stairs and running.

from the bloodstream due to the store's supply of blood to the tissue, which thereby creates heat. An amazing property! This is the same kind of heat production that you experience while running or doing other physical training. If you've been training for a period of time, you'll notice a change in your hot and cold sensation, as with increased muscle mass the body is simply better at staying warm. You can take advantage of this if you want to swim for longer, or even become an ice swimmer.

White fat

But isn't it white fat that keeps us warm? Partly, yes, but muscles are better at producing heat, while white fat acts more as insulation. White fat is stored around our inner organs, and on our abdomen, hips, buttocks and thighs. Unlike muscle, white fat has a poor supply of blood and, accordingly, poor oxygen uptake and heat production. It takes a relatively long time for a white-fat cell to be activated compared to a muscle cell. White fat stores energy, as opposed to muscle, which can burn energy quickly. So, it doesn't help your swimming performance to have little lean muscle mass and lots of white fat. In fact, a large amount of muscle mass combined with a medium amount of white fat (that is to say, something in the normal body fat percentage) can be the sweet spot.

Becoming an ice swimmer

It's good to have goals and ambitions when undertaking a new sport or lifestyle; personal goals keep you motivated. If your goal is to be an ice swimmer, you can easily do it by building up cold acclimatization.

Swimming in water below 5°C (41°F) is called "ice swimming" and is practised in most countries with cold winters. In Denmark we rarely have a lot of ice on the water, and when it comes it doesn't stay long. But there are many freshwater lakes that reach 5°C or freeze over more quickly than then sea does. Ice swimming is a sport in which you can compete on an international level. You can call yourself an ice swimmer if you are able to complete ten swimming strokes and swim twenty-five metres (twenty-seven yards) in water below 5°C. If you like, you can participate in the Ice Swimming World Championship. (However, it is recommended that you consult your GP before embarking on this mission.) Impressively, Denmark competed in Estonia in March 2018, taking fourth place out of forty countries. Denmark could well become the Nordic region's leading ice-swimming nation.

Since 2009, official ice-swimming competitions have been held around the world. The International Ice Swimming Association (IISA) was founded on 1 July 2009 by South African ice swimmer Ram Barkai in Cape Town, South Africa. On 31 January 2009, Barkai swam 2.33 kilometres (1½ miles) in forty-three minutes in water that was 4°C (39°F). It was the beginning of the famous "ice mile" (1609 metres).

Ice swimming isn't recommended for people with no experience of winter swimming before they've undergone cold acclimatization.

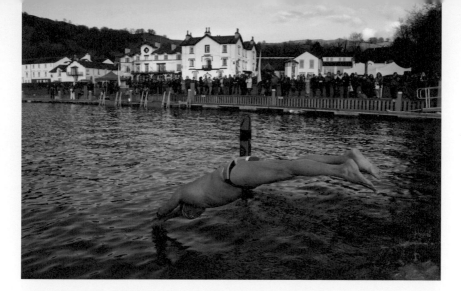

Above: Ram Barkai competing at a Chillswim open water swimming event at Lake Windermere, England.

For safety reasons, it is important to differentiate between ice-swimming athletes and non-athletes. Athletes compete at high intensity in cold water for several minutes, while non-athletes may sit in ice-cold water without physical activity. The difference in physical shape, movement in the water and hardening to the cold have a great impact on the cooling rate of the body. So, how do you start building up your ice swimming? It's a great advantage for performance to have control over your breathing. If you reduce your body fat and build muscle in the process, you can improve your cold tolerance. This is the best prognosis for positive experiences as an ice swimmer. You can do your cardio workout through weightlifting or running sessions before or after winter swimming. The combinations affect your circulatory system by improving the vasomotor function. This will help you train your body to warm up quickly.

People with heart disease are at greater risk of side effects from ice-cold water. It can cause arrhythmia and acute cardiovascular events. Therefore, a step-by-step strategy is recommended to begin and then expand the activity. Building up resistance serves the purpose of habituation and also protects against possible risks. Even if you feel your progress is slow, you will gain from the health benefits of winter swimming.

The cold shower

"One-two-three, now! . . ." No, not yet. I'm preparing myself. OK, try again . . . One-two-three, NOW!" And I turn the handle from red to blue in a single movement. My pulse is already racing from the excitement and expectation of cold water, and – "AAAARGHHH! IT'S COLD!" The body reacts violently, as if it's just waking up and the skin is screaming "WHAT IN THE WORLD ARE YOU DOING . . . WE TAKE WARM BATHS, ISN'T THAT ENOUGH!?"

If we are not acclimatized, a cold shower can feel like needles on the skin. The upper body hurts and it is a strangely mixed warm-and-cold sensation on the lower body. With quick movements I distribute both the water and the pain. My little boys have come in and are staring at me in amazement.

"Mum, what are you doing?"

Has it even been thirty seconds? No, it hasn't. I turn the water off and get out of the shower.

"Well, mummy's just taking a cold shower. It's actually really healthy," I say, but my boys don't look convinced. It probably takes practice to make it look healthy. This was my cold shower debut a few years ago. Like anyone else, I needed to build up resistance to be able to stay calm and enjoy the refreshing cold.

A way of treating physical and mental illness

In the early nineteenth century, doctors designed the first showers for the purpose of curing the mentally ill. These theories supposedly date back to the middle of the seventeenth century, when a mentally ill man was chained to an open wagon. He managed to free himself and jumped into the cold sea, whereupon he fainted. He was rescued from the water, and when he came to, he was no longer insane and lived on without experiencing further "bouts of insanity".

After this episode, cold water was considered a miracle treatment for mental illness, and doctors began to send their patients into the water. Unfortunately, many were kept (or maybe even held) in the water for

COLD FACTS:
UNDER THE COLD SHOWER

- Decide how many seconds you want to start with, and increase by five seconds each day. The first thirty seconds are the hardest but the most important. Thirty seconds for thirty days will boost your immune system.

- Prepare mentally: relax your shoulders to embrace the cold.

- Just do it: turn the hot water to cold, and move about under the shower to distribute the water over your body. Breathe and count the seconds.

- Over a period of time, try to make the water colder and colder, to habituate your body for your winter swim start-up.

- Take one in the morning and you will feel fresh and exhilarated for the rest of the day.

- To get the full benefit of the cold-shock response, avoid switching back and forth between hot and cold temperatures.

- Enjoy the tingly feeling – it feels like champagne under your skin. Once you get used to the cold, it's a great opportunity to go one step further and become a winter swimmer!

too long and died of hypothermia. Doctors believed that a heated, inflamed brain was the physical cause of mental illness, and that the water cooled it. Despite many deaths, cold showers were introduced in prisons, but eventually these too were abolished and replaced with hot baths and other hygienic measures. The (hot) shower then served to improve the health of the population and has ever since.

Cold exposure for mentally ill patients was clearly overdone in the seventeenth century. Today it is broadly known that lengthy cold exposure can be fatal, and that short exposure can be beneficial to health. But how much cold exposure is healthy? Scientific studies examining the effects of cold showers on health are lacking, but there is one clinical randomized controlled trial, conducted in 2016 in the Netherlands, which specifically tested the effects of time spent in a cold shower on health outcomes and work absenteeism. A group of 3,018 participants were randomly assigned to take a (hot to-) cold shower for 0 (control group), 30, 60 or 90 seconds for 30 days. Seventy-nine per cent took the cold showers daily for 30 days, and results showed a 29 per cent reduction in sick leave after 90 days, relative to the control group. There was no difference in sick leave if the cold showers were 30, 60 or 90 seconds long.

The effect on quality of life, work productivity, anxiety and thermal sensitivity were also compared between the groups, as well as any serious side effects. No serious side effects were reported in those taking cold showers for up to ninety seconds. In fact a slightly improved quality of life and increased energy was noted among the cold-shower groups. These are quite interesting results, but is it possible to maintain this kind of routine? It seems that 91 per cent of the participants wanted to continue cold showers after the study ended, and 64 per cent of them kept to this routine after three months. These results are impressive, but an obvious limitation of the study is that the participants cannot be ignorant of the intervention. The placebo effect can mean it's possible they will feel less ill in the knowledge they are doing something that is believed to be healthy.

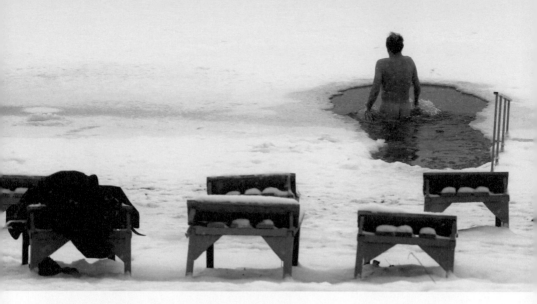

Above: Ice-hole bathing in the Dnieper river in Kyiv, Ukraine.

Several studies have investigated the effect of cold water on illness severity and sick leave. They conclude that acute cold exposure has a positive effect on the immune system and causes an increase in antioxidants that help the body defend itself against viruses. These physiological adaptations could be the explanation for fewer days off sick. You will read more about the immune system in Chapter 10 (Does It Make You Healthier?).

As discussed in Chapter 5 (The Cold-Shock Response), considering the relatively mild effect of a routine cold shower or a few seconds/minutes in cold water on hormonal and cytokine modulation, these alone are unlikely to play a significant role. Instead, it is likely explained by fast neural activation and the secretion of neurotransmitters in the brain and to the body's circulatory system. It is possible that neuroimaging technologies such as functional MRI could be used to measure a potential neurobiological immunostimulatory effect during cold exposure.

Cold adaptation in the shower

We probably all know people who end their daily shower with a blast of cold water. I have met many in the older generation, and as a child I always wondered how pain from cold could be healthy. These days

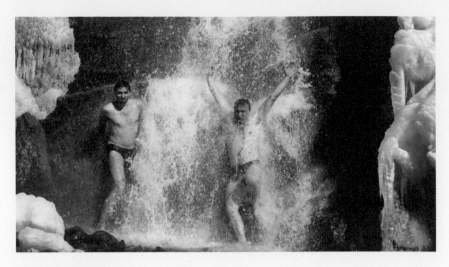

Above: The ultimate cold shower.

we have more scientific research to back up the old anecdotal stories about cold and health, and over the last few years I have been asked many times if cold showers give any of the same benefits as winter swimming.

The answer is both yes and no. A study from 2005 looked into whether repeated cold showers could be a method of habituation for cold-water immersion. Researchers investigated the relationship between temperature change to the skin and the subjects' breathing rate as an indication of habituation. Those subjects who took regular showers at 10°C (50°F) took fewer breaths than those who had showered using warmer water (15°C/59°F) when they went into cold-water tubs containing water at 10°C. This suggests that if the water temperature in the shower is the same as that of the seawater, you can habituate your body to cold water before you start winter swimming. But if the shower is just 5°C (9°F) warmer, you'll experience a cold shock. Controlling and adjusting the water temperature can be a challenge, however. Why is that?

I talked to my husband, an engineer, who happens to have a unique knowledge of water supply systems in Denmark. He informed me that

TIP: If you have an important meeting, interview or exam, taking a cold shower beforehand is a really good way to clear your head. A little boost in endorphins, adrenalin and noradrenalin will make you more energetic, positive and mentally ready for the task at hand.

in winter in the countryside, tap water temperature can reach a low of 6°C (42°F), because it stands for a long time in pipes in the cold ground. In the city, where there's greater water consumption, it will be warmer. In the summer especially, tap water is rarely below 16°C (60°F). Shower temperature can be used for habituation to cold water in general, but it is challenging to adjust according to the temperature in the sea. If you don't have access to winter swimming in open water or a water tub, cold showers are definitely a good alternative.

Cold showers versus winter swimming

There are two reasons why a cold shower cannot compare to winter swimming. The first has to do with the seasons. Habituation to open water temperatures happens gradually and in parallel with seasonal changes. Just when you think you've become habituated to the water, the water and air temperature can change suddenly, and you experience a new round of the cold-shock response. This is why it is never boring to winter swim in the Nordic countries, where nature and weather are so unpredictable – you won't find that unpredictability in the shower.

The second reason is physiological. In the shower, water hits the body in the form of droplets. The droplets mostly make contact with the upper body and are warmed by your skin as they run down your legs, sending mixed signals to your brain. In contrast, winter swimming is a whole-body cold-water immersion which triggers a response in the sympathetic nervous system as well as the diving response described in Chapter 5 (The Cold-Shock Response). Full immersion exerts hydrostatic pressure (which cold showers don't) and stimulates baroreceptors (arterial and cardiopulmonary), causing an inhibition of the sympathetic nervous system and an increase in vagal tone. This will lower heart rate and blood pressure due to parasympathetic activation. The latter also controls cortisol and serotonin levels and might be partly responsible for the health benefits observed in winter swimmers. As the diving response isn't activated during cold showers, the benefits are unlikely to be the same as with cold-water immersion.

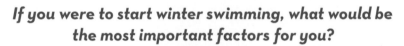

If you were to start winter swimming, what would be the most important factors for you?

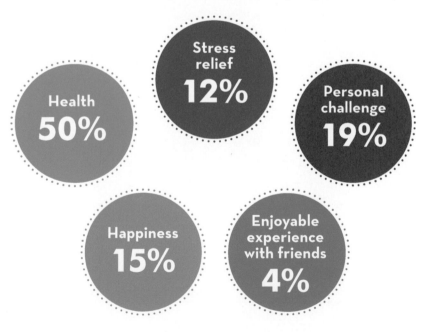

From the author's questionnaire of non-winter swimmers.

COLD FACTS:
EQUIPMENT AND PREPARATION

- Wear a swimming cap, goggles and water-repellent earplugs. You'll feel like you're in a protective bubble.

- Decide how long you want to swim before getting into the water.

- Go slowly but steadily into the water, and accept the fact that it's cold.

- Cold water has healthy energy – learn to love it!

- Learn to control your breathing and avoid panicking.

- Stay calm in the water for a minute. Take a deep breath and exhale. Repeat this until you feel ready to swim.

- Start with three to five strokes back and forth.
  You can either increase the number of strokes
  or the time spent in the water.

- A water-resistant triathlon heart-rate monitor is recommended to keep track of your heart rate, number of arm strokes and how long you've been in the water.

- A headlight is an obvious advantage in the dark.

CHAPTER 7

BROWN FAT

"Winter passes and one remembers
one's perseverance"
YOKO ONO
Artist, singer, songwriter

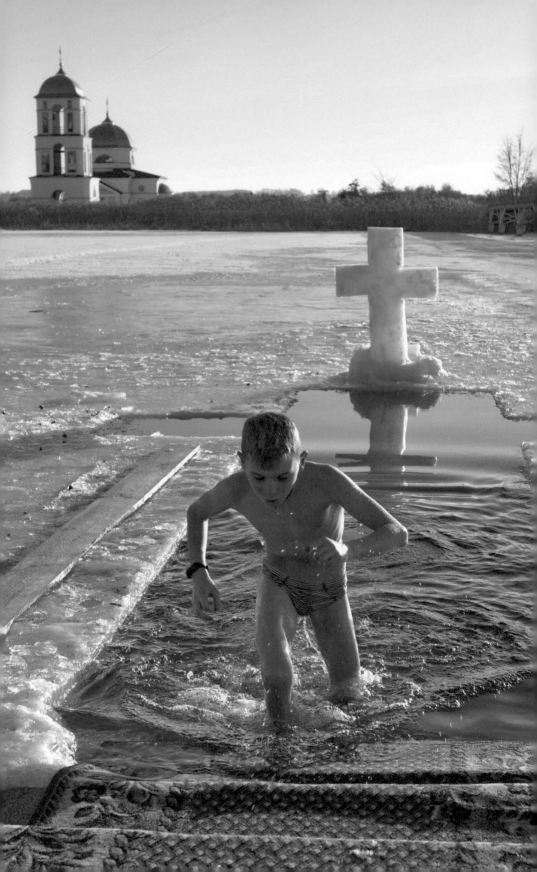

7

Brown fat is something of a wild card, and an almost unknown organ. It might sound strange that we have a kind of brown fat, in addition to the better-known white fat, but it is the reason we burn more fat when we're cold or winter swimming. The brown colour of the adipose tissue can be explained by an increased number of mitochondria in the cells, many more than in white-fat cells. Brown fat works hard for us. It keeps us healthy when we're eating, sleeping, running and cold. In fact it's working constantly.

When we're discussing the health benefits of winter swimming, one of the factors we don't yet know enough about is metabolism, i.e. fat burning. Only a few studies have tested the body's energy metabolization during cold exposure, but these are very promising. Given the obesity epidemic and the increasing prevalence of type 2 diabetes, it is worth investigating new methods and non-drug-related solutions to the problem. Maybe something as simple as the cold can help improve the situation by activating brown fat.

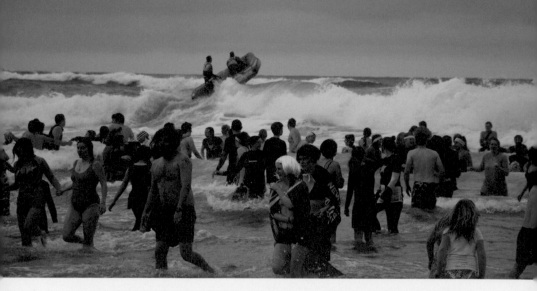

Above: The annual midwinter Polar Plunge held at St Clair Esplanade, Dunedin, New Zealand.

Page 116: In the Orthodox Church, the faithful of all ages dip three times into ice holes blessed by a priest, and often cut in the shape of a cross, at Epiphany on 19 January.

A universal problem

In the USA alone there are more than 29 million people with diabetes caused by an unhealthy lifestyle. Nearly 86 million more people are pre-diabetic. There's an incredible number of people with an increased risk of cardiovascular disease and early death due to the consequences of poor blood-sugar regulation. The primary cause of this is a surplus energy intake leading to being overweight with excessive storing of white fat. White fat is mainly located subcutaneously, around the internal organs and in the liver and muscles. It is spread throughout the body and can increase inflammation, making us ill when there's too much of it. Fat deposits can grow so large that the fat percentage exceeds blood, water, muscle and bone.

This is a reality for many people. We know that white fat sends signals in the body, as if "talking" with the internal organs, and with the brain in particular. If the white fat becomes a large and dominating element, it can have too much influence.

The causes of diabetes are still being researched, but decreased insulin sensitivity is generally considered to be the primary cause of blood-sugar imbalance. How so? Whether you develop diabetes or not depends on how sensitive your cells are to insulin and the ability to produce insulin in the pancreas. When cells don't recognize insulin, it isn't absorbed, resulting in elevated levels of sugar in the blood, which in turn results in diabetes. There's a subsequent cascade of consequences and conditions, including increased fat deposits in blood vessels, which increases the risk of clotting, neuropathy, numbness in fingers and toes, legs and hands, along with impaired vision. Ultimately, it decreases the number of healthy years a person has, and affects quality of life and life expectancy. If this is your current situation or that of someone you know, you need to know that you can do something about it.

Even the smallest changes in lifestyle can have a significant impact on your health. Current research is looking for new solutions – preferably even before the problems begin. Scientists are exploring new ways to increase the cells' sensitivity to insulin, and increased energy expenditure is critical to this. Insulin sensitivity then improves, and cells are able to remove sugar from the bloodstream, as well as absorb sugar and fat from stores in the body and use them as energy. This is how the body loses weight.

Why are we still discussing the weight-loss equation? We already know what works: diet, exercise and medical intervention. All this is true, but we should never stop looking for alternative treatment methods, particularly when we see increasing obesity in the world. The current solutions are obviously not keeping up with the problem.

Let's keep medical intervention out of the discussion for the moment, to consider more fully the specific lifestyle changes that increase metabolism. Diet and exercise have shown beneficial effects in the treatment of diabetes, but a number of studies have also indicated that exposure to cold may have positive effects on insulin sensitivity. This is where your brown fat comes in.

COLD FACTS:
WHAT IS TYPE 2 DIABETES?

Definition from the World Health Organization:
"Diabetes is a chronic, metabolic disease characterized by elevated levels of blood glucose (or blood sugar), which leads over time to serious damage to the heart, blood vessels, eyes, kidneys and nerves. The most common is type 2 diabetes, usually in adults, which occurs when the body becomes resistant to insulin or doesn't make enough insulin."

- Over the past three decades, the prevalence of type 2 diabetes has increased dramatically in all countries and at all income levels. There's a global agreement towards a goal of ending the increase of diabetes and obesity before 2025.

- The number of people with diabetes rose from 108 million in 1980 to 422 million in 2014.

- The global prevalence of diabetes among adults increased from 4.7 per cent in 1980 to 8.5 per cent in 2014.

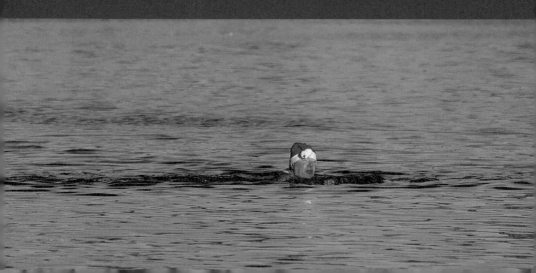

Pre-diabetes can be detected with a fasting blood test that identifies a reduced ability to absorb sugar from the bloodstream into the cells, resulting in elevated blood-sugar levels during fasting. People with pre-diabetes have a high risk of developing type 2 diabetes, but can avoid it with lifestyle changes that have been shown to be effective in preventing or delaying diabetes:

- Achieve and maintain a healthy body weight.

- Engage in physical activity for at least thirty minutes every day, with moderate intensity on most days.

- Maintain a healthy diet with a minimum of sugar and saturated fat.

- Abstain from tobacco – smoking increases the risk of diabetes and cardiovascular diseases.

Below: Swimmers participate in the annual Christmas winter swimming competition in the Vltava river, Prague, Czech Republic.

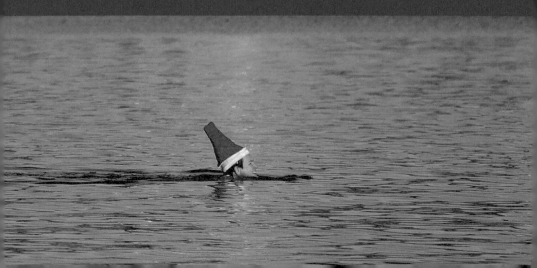

What is brown fat?

Brown fat was first documented in 1551 by the naturalist Conrad Gessner, who described an organ found in marmots "which was neither muscle nor fat, but something in between", and that was "brown". Is brown fat really brown? Well, you could say it's brown-ish, since it was originally identified solely by its colour. As mentioned earlier, 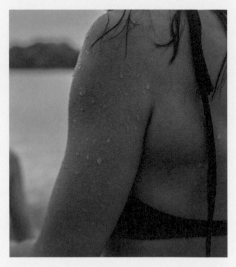 the colour is due to the fat's granular and mitochondrial (the cell's energy powerhouse and metabolism engine) content. A brown-fat cell contains triglycerides, a nucleus and a lot of mitochondria. When the brown-fat cell is activated, the mitochondria split the fat inside the cell with the production of adenosine triphosphate (ATP) – a molecule that carries energy within cells – and the energy is released directly as heat in the body. To create that energy, the brown-fat cells pull sugar and fat from the bloodstream as fuel. Brown fat is unique because it can be activated to burn energy and produce heat in a process that goes like this: cold temperatures are detected on the skin, which signals via nerves to the brain. Noradrenalin is released and activates the brown-fat cells to perform a mechanism called thermogenesis – heat production. Thermogenesis takes place in the mitochondria of the brown-fat cells.

Until fifteen or twenty years ago, brown fat was thought to be a merely insignificant tissue in adults. Scientists believed that it existed in large proportions only in newborns, where it was important for maintaining a sufficiently high core temperature, as muscle shivering is not developed in the infant state. Historically, it was also believed that the tissue disappeared as a person got older, until the 1970s when it was discovered during PET/CT scanning of adults. There may have been earlier pieces of evidence that were neglected, but the rediscovery was exciting news. The question then arises: What is the purpose of brown fat in adults? It must have important functions; otherwise, evolutionarily, we would have lost it.

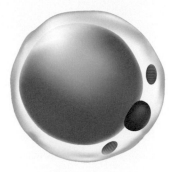 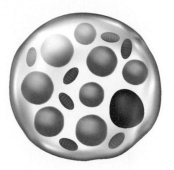

White fat
In the centre of the cell is a large droplet of lipid/fat (triglyceride). The nucleus (shown above in purple) and mitochondria are therefore very close to the edge of the cell, which means it is difficult for the mitochondria to create energy. Fat burn is slow.

Brown fat
Each cell contains numerous smaller lipid droplets and more mitochondria, which are spread out, and therefore produce energy more rapidly. Fat and sugar is taken from the bloodstream as fuel for energy production.

The largest deposits detected by PET/CT scanning were found to be located around the neck (collarbone) and along the spine, while smaller deposits were noticed around the heart and kidneys. At that time, it was thought that brown fat played a role in the thermoregulation of blood to and from the brain. With that definition its function was considered a vital one, that of maintaining our brain at a steady temperature when we get cold. PET/CT scans are still considered the best method for identifying brown fat, and for brown fat to be visible in a scan, it must be activated. And what activates the sympathetic nervous system? A winter swimmer would know the answer – the cold! Cold is the fastest and most effective "activator". During a PET/CT scan, a specific radioactive sugar called fluorodeoxyglucose

(FDG) is injected into a blood vessel and stores itself in metabolically active tissue – i.e. the brown fat. Because brown fat uses sugar from the bloodstream as fuel when it is active, the brown fat takes in the radioactive sugar. The sugar stays in the brown-fat cells for a short time and is then visible in the PET/CT scan. The FDG is then excreted in urine. You need a specialized scanning device, cold temperatures and a radioactive sugar to see brown fat – the entire process/method is abbreviated as FDG-PET/CT.

How does the cold activate brown fat?

Receptors in the skin sense the cold and activate the sympathetic nervous system. The signal is sent to the temperature-regulating centre in the hypothalamus, which increases neural noradrenalin release. Noradrenalin attaches to specific beta-receptors on the surface of brown-fat cells, which triggers the release of ATP (energy) and heat. This activation cascade is rapid and part of the cold-shock response.

Since the rediscovery, the presence of brown fat has been confirmed in biopsies taken from both mice and humans. We know that we have brown fat, but many questions remain unanswered because research into brown fat is still in the early stages. We would like to know more about who has it and whether winter swimming can impact our brown fat function by repeated stimulation.

Can the cold create more brown fat?

In scientific experiments, hypotheses are often first tested on animals. If evidence suggests a similarity with humans, research goes a step further. That's why there have been a number of studies on rodents and humans which have provided evidence that the cold activates brown fat and creates more of the tissue, increases energy metabolism and improves insulin sensitivity and blood-sugar balance. This is good news, and we now know that brown fat not only keeps us warm, but

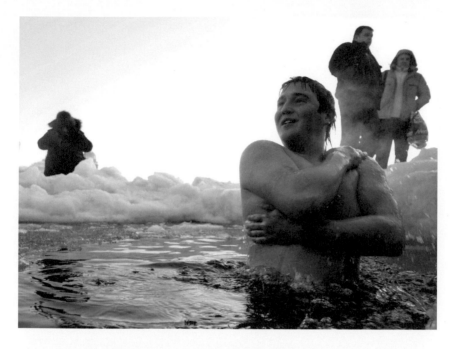

Above: It is believed that the ritual of plunging into ice water at Epiphany brings strength, good health and joy for the year ahead.

also possesses health-promoting properties. Researchers working on brown fat are on a mission to figure out how to promote these benefits in a way that makes sense. Let's look more closely at the evidence of continuous cold exposure.

In one study of middle-aged women who swam in cold water for an entire season, an increased sensitivity to insulin was found, which could mean that cold water has long-term effects on balancing blood sugar. The study did not determine if the improvements were related to brown fat, but in their report the researchers raised the question of whether brown fat may be the cause.

Another study examined the effect of continuous cold room temperature on brown fat activity and the amount of brown fat, to explore whether people develop more brown fat by sleeping in cool rooms. Adult subjects slept for one month in a room with a room temperature of 24°C (74°F), and FDG-PET/CT scans revealed that they had very little brown fat. Then the same people slept for a month in a room kept at 19°C (66°F), and new scans revealed a marked increase in brown fat quantities. The following month they once again slept in 24°C, with the result that the proportion of the brown fat had once again decreased. For the fourth and final month of the experiment, they slept in a room kept at 27°C (80°F) and found that their brown fat disappeared almost entirely. Moreover, in the cold month the subjects showed improved insulin sensitivity.

The study thus confirms that persistent exposure to cold can help to create greater quantities of brown fat and improve insulin sensitivity, and others confirm similar results. One study of subjects with diabetes or obesity equipped them with cooling vests at a temperature of 14–15°C (59–60°F), which they wore for ten days. A before-and-after FDG-PET/CT scan revealed that they all showed an increase in their brown fat. They also had improved cellular insulin sensitivity.

In another study in which subjects each sat by an open window for half an hour for twenty consecutive days, they too showed an increase in brown fat. Each of these studies used different cooling methods, but all show an improvement in insulin sensitivity, which can potentially regulate blood-sugar balance. It is not known, however, to what extent the improvements are due to muscle versus brown fat activity.

Both the amount of brown fat and how active it is will determine how much energy it can burn while a person is cold. It's quite amazing that the body has a healthy kind of fat that gets activated by cold and can be used to access our sugar and fat stores. First, the brown fat burns sugar and fat from the bloodstream, which will then release lipids from white-fat stores and sugar from liver and muscle stores. Unlike white fat, brown fat is activated incredibly quickly when exposed to the cold

Opposite: Winter, Oulu, Finland – air temperature -24°C (-11°F), water 3°C (37°F)

and burns energy straightaway. Studies have found that if you put a hand or a foot in a bucket of iced water, you'll activate brown fat in seconds or minutes, and this is detectable on PET/CT scans. This is not the case with white fat, unfortunately.

It is exciting that we are able to influence the amount of brown fat we store in our bodies, and thereby affect our health. Think about it as having an internal wood-burning stove that burns energy even when you're not running or exercising – and even when you're not cold. Brown fat is an extra "calorie eater" that contributes to the bottom line when it comes to energy expenditure. But we don't yet know if we have found a good, feasible way to activate brown fat, or whether this is possible by winter swimming.

Brown fat and winter swimming

So, let's reflect on our findings. We could just start recommending that people wear cooling vests, sleep in a room at 19°C (66°F), take cold footbaths, or sit by an open window for twenty minutes every day when it's cold outside. It's not attractive, though, nor convenient or practical to walk around in public in a cooling vest. Nor is it considerate to lower the heat in a home you're sharing with other household members. That's not to say that it wouldn't be a good idea to drop the heat a bit from 24 to 22°C (75 to 71°F). Similarly, it could be

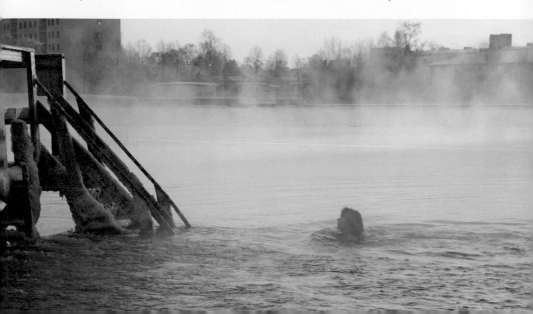

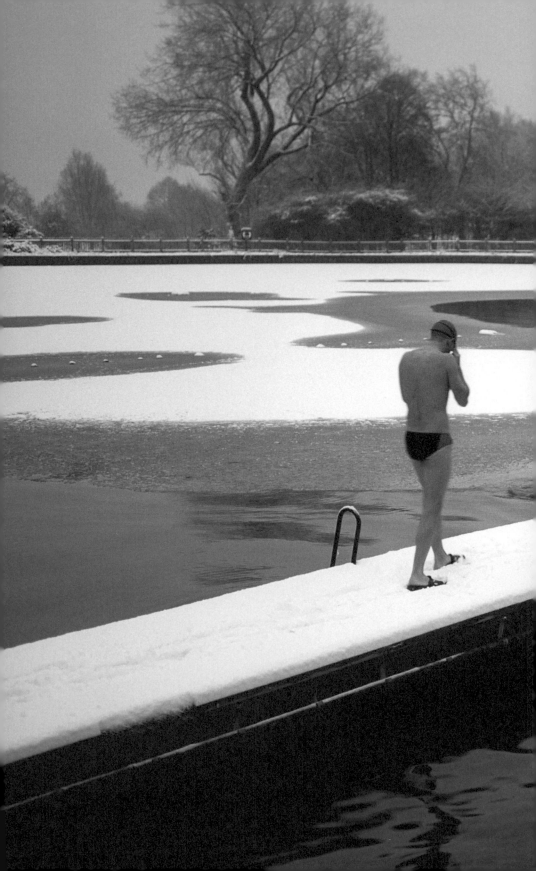

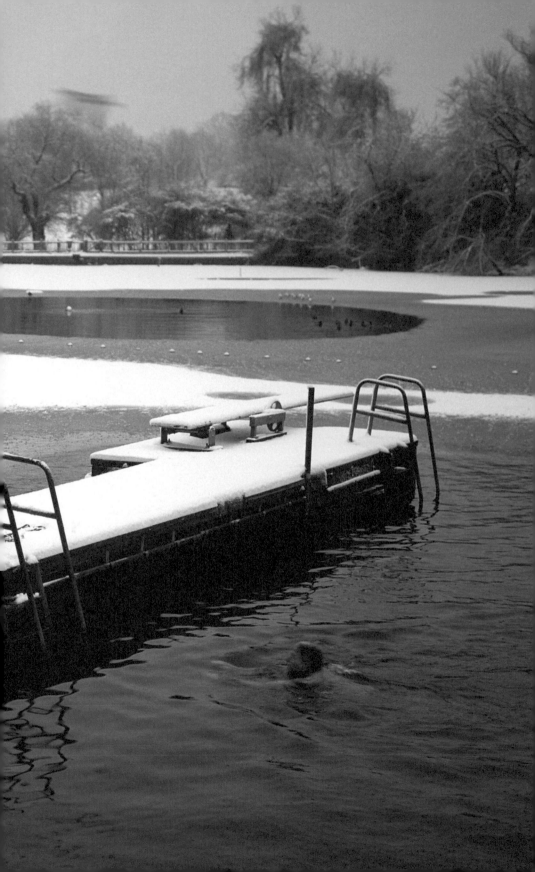

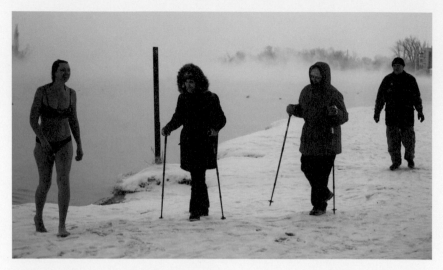

Above: A river bank near Moscow, Russia.

Pages 128–129: Highgate Men's Pond at Hampstead Heath, London, England.

recommended that people sleep in a room that's a little cooler than the living room. Apart from these living modifications to increase your brown fat, what are the alternatives?

If you can generate more brown fat from sleeping in the cold or wearing cooling vests, it's conceivable that regular winter swimming would increase the amount of this tissue in our bodies to an even greater extent. This could be attributable to several things, both behavioural and physiological: the direct positive effect of cold water, which stimulates a cascade of neurotransmitters and hormones in the body, motivating people to swim again and again for the pure thrill of it. It gets people moving and out into the cold, which activates the sympathetic nervous system. When you immerse yourself in cold water, noradrenalin rises dramatically, up to 180 per cent above basal levels within two minutes. The level drops quickly when you get out of the water again. Studies have shown that the sudden and intense cooling of the skin accounts for the dramatic increase in noradrenalin which, as explained earlier, activates the brown fat.

We still know too little about how much brown fat humans have and how many calories are burned during cooling, even after a brief plunge in the water. It would be interesting to measure the long-term effects of winter swimming on brown fat for a full season, and in fact this is the subject of my PhD studies. We are currently working on the results for publication.

Why do we have brown fat?

We're born with brown fat, and newborns have, proportionately speaking, quite a bit of brown fat between the shoulder blades. The amount of brown fat in adults is difficult to determine exactly, but it is estimated to be between 200 and 1500 grams (7 and 53 ounces), while some adults have none left or never had any in the first place. Studies have shown that the amount of brown fat decreases with age, and we need to activate it in order to keep it. Maybe we should think of it in the same way we think of building muscle: you invest time and energy in activating it, and improve your health a little every day.

It is interesting to note what happens with our brown fat between our infant state and old age. When newborns under six months begin to get cold, their muscles don't yet have the ability to contract, and so they cannot keep themselves warm by shivering. Scientists believe that the evolutionary purpose of brown fat is to produce heat in newborns when they get cold, ensuring or at least increasing their chances of survival.

Today it may seem unnecessary to talk about brown fat as vital, if we consider how comfortably most of us live in terms of temperature, and how infants are unlikely to freeze in our heated and fully insulated homes. Do we really need brown fat, one may ask? Despite the extra heat we enjoy from warm houses and clothing, man as a species has managed to retain this lightning-fast heating tissue.

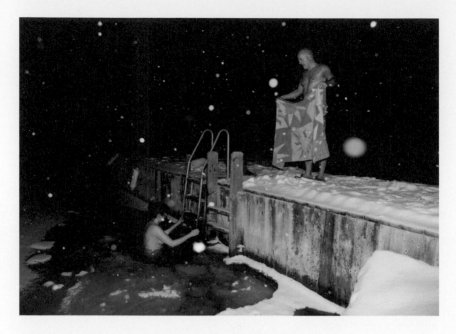

Above: A dry towel to look forward to, Stockholm, Sweden.

As we grow to adulthood, the amount of brown fat we have decreases. This is probably due to the larger surface area of our bodies, which produces fewer temperature fluctuations. The body gets better at maintaining a stable temperature, which may remove the primary function of brown fat and cause it to decrease in size. It may even disappear entirely.

Surprisingly, studies show that most healthy and normal-weight adults under the age of forty still have deposits of brown fat. This is very good news, as it means there's hope that we can enlist help from this calorie-consuming organ, even as adults, especially as we risk becoming overweight with age. After the age of forty something interesting happens when it comes to energy expenditure, but not in a positive way. Many functions in the body change noticeably – and first and foremost our ability to burn energy diminishes. Many people notice that the usual run isn't enough to keep the weight off. This is unfortunate as people become more busy with children and their careers, and perhaps have more money for the finer things in life. Some people experience existential crises around middle age and are challenged in different ways, just as our ability to burn energy declines. We have less time to invest in exercise and our health, and yet our desire to kick back and enjoy life is greater.

Research has shown that people with diabetes and obesity in particular are most likely not to have much brown fat left – and many have none at all. It is also possible that the disappearance of brown fat is a reason for weight gain and a slowing metabolism. This is probably a chicken-and-egg kind of question, and the answer can't be found in this book. But every rule has exceptions. I have noted in my own experiments that some adults over the age of forty do have brown fat, including those who are both overweight and have diabetes. We don't know the reasons for this, or how it develops differently. Theories, however, point to contexts such as genetics, lifestyle and environment. If you spend a lot of time outdoors in cold temperatures or in changing weather conditions, or live in a cold country, then you probably have a higher chance of retaining brown fat through adulthood. Consistent activation of brown fat is probably needed in order to maintain it.

Brown fat in practice

White fat is not all bad – in fact, it's deeply needed; dysfunction of the white fat storage in your body would make you very ill. You need what we may call a "small energy bank". But it can also be detrimental if that bank gets too big. White fat stores energy in the body, while brown fat mainly expends energy. Repeated exposure to cold gives brown fat greater activation and higher energy expenditure. In my studies we hypothesized that repeated exposure to cold water increases the activation of brown fat. It could also be the cold-shock response that activates brown fat, as previously mentioned. As a result, we believe that cold swimming will increase energy metabolization, improve insulin sensitivity and possibly also lower blood sugar in people whose energy metabolism is disturbed. To measure possible improvements in these areas, we've tested them in overweight people over forty years of age who have pre-diabetes.

Pre-diabetes means that a person's blood-sugar levels lie in a grey zone between normal and high, when they will be diagnosed with type 2 diabetes. It can be difficult to detect diabetes in its early stages, as it is often largely asymptomatic.

However, if you are fortunate enough to discover that your blood-sugar levels are in the grey zone, there is a great deal you can do to change direction and bring your blood sugar down. It is no surprise that you need to exercise!

A number of people with blood-sugar readings in the grey zone signed up for our trial, hoping that winter swimming would help their condition by increasing energy metabolism, and for the enjoyment of it too, of course.

When they were recruited, many of our subjects asked: "Brown fat, what's that? Isn't this about winter swimming?"

"Yes, of course it is," I would reply. "But there's more to the story. Brown fat is the underlying motivation for the project. If we can increase energy expenditure by activating our brown fat through winter swimming, we might increase the function even when we are not exercising." If the existing brown fat can be activated, or if we can create more brown fat, it might be possible to burn excess white fat even faster and for longer, only with cold. One day we may find a biomarker that can do just that. But we need to learn more about secreted factors from the brown fat, and differences and similarities between the two types of adipose tissue and how they affect each other.

Not brown, not white – but beige!

Research from the past decade has shown that cells in white adipose tissue can be transformed into something similar to brown-fat cells when exposed to cold environments, and in this way can attain properties like those of brown adipose tissue. The new cells are called "beige", and the process "browning". It may be that browning can occur with cold exposure by winter swimming, wearing a cooling vest, sitting at an open window, taking cold showers, sleeping in a cold room or by chemical means. Just as brown fat can be activated with cold, it may be possible to chemically activate white-fat cells to form beige-fat cells. From experiments we know that beige-fat cells remain in the same spoturge in the white adipose tissue but have the ability to burn faster than their neighbouring white-fat cells. Browning can thus reduce obesity and the risk of diabetes, and scientists are working to find ways to increase browning in our body.

Brown fat in a bottle

Over the past few years, several studies have focused on activating brown fat to increase energy expenditure. But little is known about how brown fat communicates with other organs and affects functions in the body. It is likely that brown fat, when activated, sends out various healthy signals called "batokines", which can activate functions in other organs. For example, brown fat might send out batokines to increase browning, or to lessen appetite by signalling to the appetite control centre in the brain. It is certainly a popular research area, as the batokines could help to combat lifestyle diseases. Until we know more, we will simply enjoy the natural health benefits of winter swimming and cold-activated brown fat.

CHAPTER 8

ON YOUR OWN OR WITH A CLUB?

"You can't buy happiness. BUT . . . you can swim in the cold sea with your friends and drink hot chocolate with marshmallows, and that's kind of the same thing"
SUSANNA SØBERG

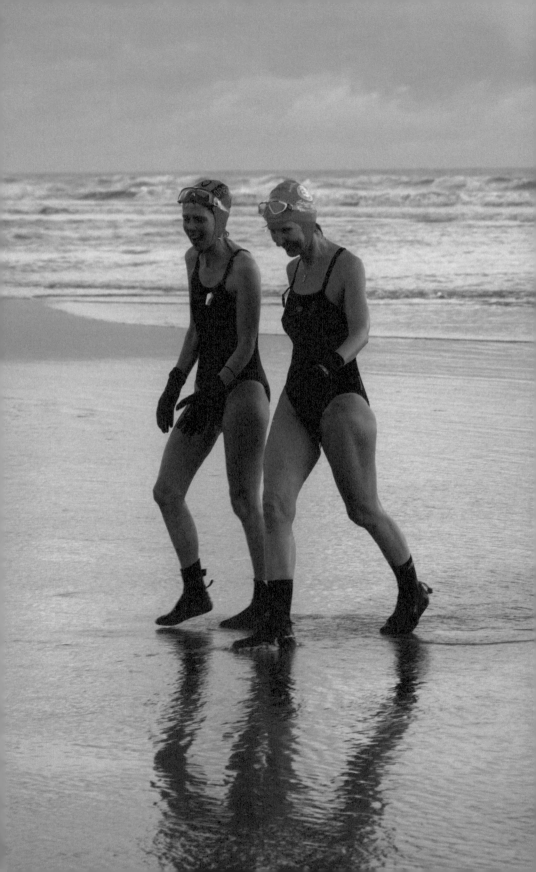

8

*More and more people are keen to start winter swimming
these days. More people, in fact, than swimming clubs
have room for. People who haven't yet started winter
swimming say that they would prefer to join a club, which
will in itself provide them with the motivation to begin.
Unfortunately, the shortage of clubs and membership
for new winter swimmers is one of the biggest barriers to
getting started. For some clubs in Denmark you have to
be on a waiting list for years, and at others you've got to
be ready to sign up online on a given day.*

The oasis of the club

Many winter swimmers talk about clubs very positively, some as their
"oasis", where they come several times a week - or even several times
a day! I was lucky enough, along with my research subjects, to get
temporary membership to a winter swimming club in Copenhagen.
A small group of women I often see in the club lounge told me that
they arrange to meet there before and after swimming. Their routine
was to go in the water, and then to the sauna. Afterwards they have
a cup of coffee in the lounge. People find or form groups here, and

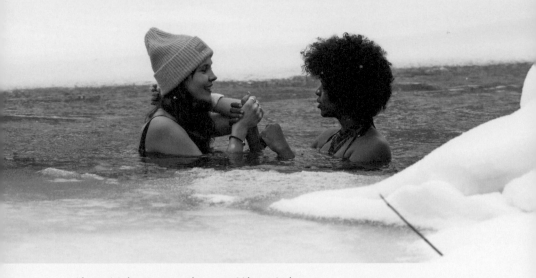

Above: Midwinter togetherness, Vilnius, Lithuania.

Page 138: Camaraderie at Brighton Beach, England.

many become friends and meet outside the club too. But some of the people in my other studies just swam off the jetty with some friends, instead of waiting for membership.

Community and togetherness

If I hadn't been fortunate enough to have the opportunity to be a club member for a season, I wouldn't have understood what's so special about it. The camaraderie, the culture, it's so open and positive – and it's certainly infectious. You look forward to going out and swimming, having a sauna afterwards and meeting other people – and you go home even happier. This happiness is a combination of "post-swimming high", as we might call the rush that the body gets as part of the cold-shock response, and the pleasure we get from being around other people, where there's no peer pressure. It's a stress-free zone, and it's something staff and members cherish. And there are rules – both practical and social – which serve to maintain the positive and relaxed atmosphere. In some clubs there's a so-called "greeting duty", meaning that everyone is required to greet other members on the jetty or in the club lounge. There's respect for the quiet of the sauna, and there's space for talking and hanging out in the lounge, which is for all age groups.

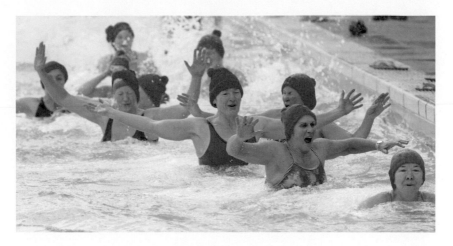

Above: Club culture at Tooting Bec Lido, London, England

Club culture

Most clubs in Denmark have an introductory meeting on site, before you start. Among other things, you're given safety instructions, for example where to find defibrillators, personal flotation devices and so on. But the club's values are also communicated, among them the strong recommendation that members leave their worries outside. This helps members to relax, and to consider the club as a haven, away from the hustle and bustle of everyday life.

In Finnish culture the sauna is used, among other things, as a kind of social icebreaker with guests before dinner, or for business people before important meetings. It is a setting for social activity where conversation is normal, while in Denmark the tendency is to be quiet so that people can meditate or reflect inwardly. Both approaches encourage positive mental health and calm, and implicit in the activity is that you leave titles and hierarchy at the door, so people can relax and be themselves. Everyone is simply a human being in the sauna. It creates an open atmosphere, and promotes a calm and positive energy similar to the culture at swimming clubs in Denmark. While not everyone knows every single person in the larger clubs, the same social rules apply, by greeting and accepting each other as we are.

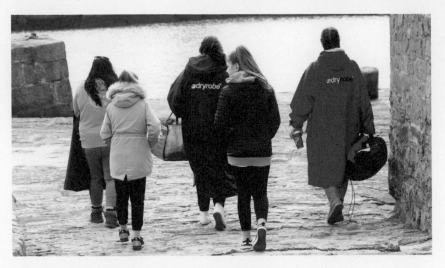

Above: The road to the sea at Porthleven, Cornwall, England.

All roads lead to the sea

But isn't it just as healthy to swim from a jetty with some friends? Yes, of course it is, and I've met a great many winter swimmers who do just that. They might be meeting anyway, to work out, run or do some other activity, and end the session with a dip in the cold water. People who live close to the sea often take a swift dip before going to work. Access to a sauna, along with the community and the lounge, are the main attractions of a club membership, but facilities such as changing rooms and showers also count. This is partly being solved in Denmark as more mobile saunas are being set up in various places.

Nudity

Many people wonder whether winter swimming should be undertaken with or without swimwear. In Denmark it's largely a question of preference, but some clubs have rules. Over the last couple of years I've come to understand why many winter swimmers swim naked: it's actually too cold with the swimsuit, and it diminishes the experience of being in the water and getting out again. The full benefit of the cold-shock response and the subsequent warming happens best if the body isn't in any doubt. The cold, wet bathing suit gives mixed signals to the brain as it's still icy cold, and it holds on to the water. The body reacts as if it's still exposed to the cold, and it's hard to warm up as all blood vessels in the body continue to contract. Without a swimsuit your skin dries and the body warms up faster as the brain receives the information to relax.

Nudity is practical, too, as swimsuits are not allowed in most saunas in Scandinavia. You'd have to put on your ice-cold swimsuit again after the sauna – and it's not a great experience, trust me. It sticks to your feet and your skin and won't sit properly – your fingers stiffen and shake – you trip and stumble – AAAAARGHHH! – Yes, that's an experience from one of my first times in the water. A friend of mine, an experienced swimmer, had brought me along. After the sauna she went back out – naked – on her way to the water. She looked over her shoulder to see if I was following but I was nowhere near her, stumbling around in my bathing suit.

"Are you coming or are you having second thoughts?" she teased.

"I'm just putting on my bathing suit!" It stuck to my skin like glue. Everyone was watching, or at least that's how it felt. I caught up with her, though my experiment with the swimsuit in the cold wind had activated the cold-shock response, and I hadn't even been in the water. I was shivering like an aspen leaf as I went down the steps. Taking my swimsuit off and putting it on again wasn't the smartest idea when I knew I could only stay in the water for a few seconds.

Some female swimmers from my studies also wore a swimsuit. It worked better for them although, as with me, not optimally going in and out of the sauna. Most were brave – or impatient – and discarded their bathing suit after their first attempt at putting it on in the cold. Many chose to swim in the women's area, and so had no issue swimming naked. Some clubs in Denmark offer gender segregation, but most clubs do not, and people either just swim in suits or turn away in modesty.

It may be that nudity is more of an issue at the beginning for untrained winter swimmers, especially for women. It can be intimidating to go out naked, but with time it gets less embarrassing, and people focus on enjoying the water, the nature and the effects of the cold. Experienced winter swimmers report that being naked gives them more freedom to move, and that they feel more connected with the water and nature. In clubs in Denmark where gender segregation isn't possible, you simply get used to wearing a bathing suit and the experience of winter swimming is still wonderful. You have to do what's right for you – whether that's conquering your shyness and swimming naked, or keeping a swimsuit on in order to be able to relax and enjoy the experience.

One winter's day I was sitting in the club's cosy little lounge. There was a long table, and someone had lit tea candles. I'd gone into the lounge to wait for some of the women taking part in my study, having decided to join them for a swim. I'd made myself a cup of tea in the kitchen and sat down at the table with my cup, swimsuit and towel. Three elderly women sat a couple of chairs away. They had wet hair, so I guessed they'd been for their swim. They sat enjoying a cup of tea, and two of them were knitting as they talked. You could tell they knew each other well. At the other end of the lounge were some younger swimmers, in their twenties. Some were working on their laptops, a couple talked quietly together. Two men were looking out of the large window and discussing the weather – the frost was coming in a few days, and with it the possibility of swimming in ice – in "slush-ice", as they call it. It's supposed to be a very special experience.

"Do you prefer to swim in a bathing suit?" one of the older ladies addressed me. "Um, yeah, I'm not quite brave enough yet to get rid of it," I said, a little embarrassed about being so shy, as if I had more to hide than they did.

"It's wonderfully liberating to realize that no-one is watching you out there. Our bodies are natural, and over time you find that you don't care," said another lady.

I nodded. It had to be true, because outside the window I saw only

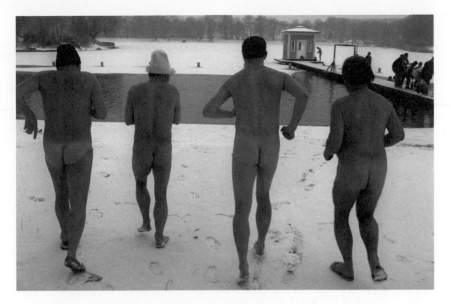

Above: Bare-faced cheek at the lido Orankesee, Berlin, Germany.

naked swimmers – young as well as old. Now it struck me that I hadn't even thought of them as naked, or even looked at them. They were just winter swimmers, and it was natural in this scenario. Men seem to be more relaxed when it comes to nudity, however. In one club in Copenhagen, there's a common area with changing rooms, sauna and bathing jetties as well as sections for women and men only, with the same facilities. But the men-only section is not as well frequented as the women's area. Most men use the common areas and are less hesitant as far as nudity is concerned.

The disappearing penis

On a cold day in October, I joined some swimmers and a novice for his first dip in the sea. He was talking a lot and was obviously very excited. "We'd better get started," he said. He also seemed nervous, so it was important to get it over with. Everyone hurried to change and he emerged naked, just like the other men and women. It was his first time but the nudity didn't seem to worry him. Not that he mentioned, at least. He was focused on the cold water and the impending first icy plunge of his life. They went down the steps and I kept watch, ready to rescue him if necessary. I cheered and guided them from the jetty. Like many others taking their first winter plunge, he was gasping out loud and thrashing around in the water. It wasn't long before he was on his way up the steps again. "MY PENIS HAS DISAPPEEEARRRED!" he shouted as he came up onto the jetty with the others. We all laughed; it was pretty amusing. It shows that both men and women are conscious of their nudity; you can overcome the embarrassment, but still it takes courage and it's a mental challenge. There is a natural resistance to undressing in public, but nudity is more accepted as part of winter swimming in the great outdoors in Denmark. It's the context and the culture of the environment you're in that makes it normal.

Finding the motivation

I'm looking out of the window and should be setting off . . . but oh, it looks cold outside – it's dark, too, and my bike's actually parked at the station . . . where's the car . . . oh no, my husband's taken it today . . . I guess I'll have to run, or walk, or take the other bike . . . yeah, good idea . . . no, it rattles too much . . . what should I do? I REALLY DON'T FEEL LIKE IT! There's also leftover cake from yesterday . . .

The above could very well be one of my streams of consciousness, which run from having a good idea all the way to the graveyard of my good intentions to stay healthy. What do you do when you just don't have the energy and it's cold outside? Here are seven tips on how to maintain your motivation.

GOOD HABITS

Sometimes it can be hard to motivate yourself, and this happens to everyone, regardless of which new endeavours you're engaging in. That's why it's important to think it through from the very beginning. What should your strategy be? We are creatures of habit, so create some good habits for yourself. Maybe you could have a winter swimming bag with all your equipment in, and towels that you can quickly swap out when you get home. A pre-packed bag is practical and makes it easier to get going. Choose a time of day that suits you best, or plan one week ahead – and put it in your calendar!

SWIM BUDDIES

Next, it's good to find a swim buddy, or preferably several you can meet up with. It's a fun challenge to take on with your friends, and then you're not swimming alone, either. You can also ask any other winter swimmers you meet on the jetty, beach or poolside. Or team up with someone at the swimming club, if you're lucky enough to be a member of one.

BE TENACIOUS

It can be hard to keep at it if you hit a few small bumps in the road and your expectations aren't completely met. Small obstacles can often cause people to give up on their goals of, for example, shedding that extra weight or sticking with winter swimming. It is perfectly normal to experience some small setbacks along the way and skip a couple of sessions, maybe more. You should not consider these a defeat, but rather a pause; you shouldn't stop winter swimming just because you missed a week or two. The body remembers the cold shock for a very long time, as brutal as that sounds, but that means that you won't be starting again at square one. Instead of giving up, arrange to meet up with your swim buddy again. Until winter swimming has become part of your lifestyle and habituation occurs, you'll need to plan and be tenacious.

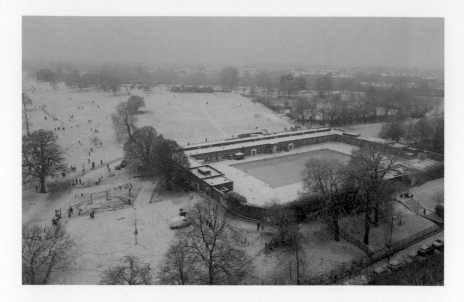

Above: Brockwell Lido, London, taken from a nearby tower block.

SPREAD THE WORD

Tell people about your plans and your accomplishments
in winter swimming. It's a good idea to invite your friends,
colleagues and family. Then you'll be accountable and it will
encourage you to continue.

TRACK YOUR PROGRESS

It's always a good idea to track your time in the water. To begin
with, you can train by counting to five or ten and gradually
increase. From my studies, I've had good experiences using
a waterproof triathlon watch with a heart-rate monitor. You
can track progress via an app, which is very motivating. Some
people take a note of the changing temperatures displayed at
the pool or club each time they go.

SET SPECIFIC AND REALISTIC GOALS

Your goal should be specific. Instead of "go winter swimming",

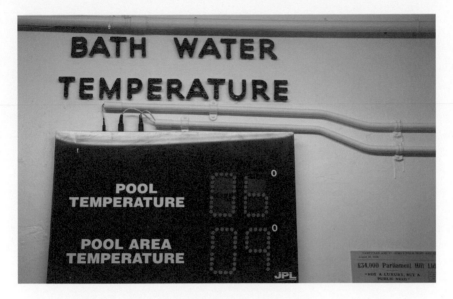

BATH WATER TEMPERATURE

POOL TEMPERATURE

POOL AREA TEMPERATURE

JPL

£54,000 Parliament Hill Lid

Above: Temperature data at Parliament Hill Lido, London.

set a goal like "go winter swimming once a week for the first three weeks". After that you can increase the goal and potentially add how many times you want to plunge at each session, or how many lengths or minutes you want to swim for. And make sure your goals are realistic. Instead of aiming to go in no time from the sofa to swimming in ice-filled water as a competitive swimmer, give yourself smaller milestones. It could be to swim twice a week for the winter season. Then progress with new goals, for example more swims or even ice swimming.

KNOW YOUR WEAKNESSES

These could be many, as people have different barriers. Maybe you get painfully cold feet or fingers. The solution might be quite simple, such as getting yourself some neoprene swim shoes and gloves. Most people bring tea or another hot drink in a Thermos, to warm their hands and to have while they're getting changed. Some also pack a hot-water bottle.

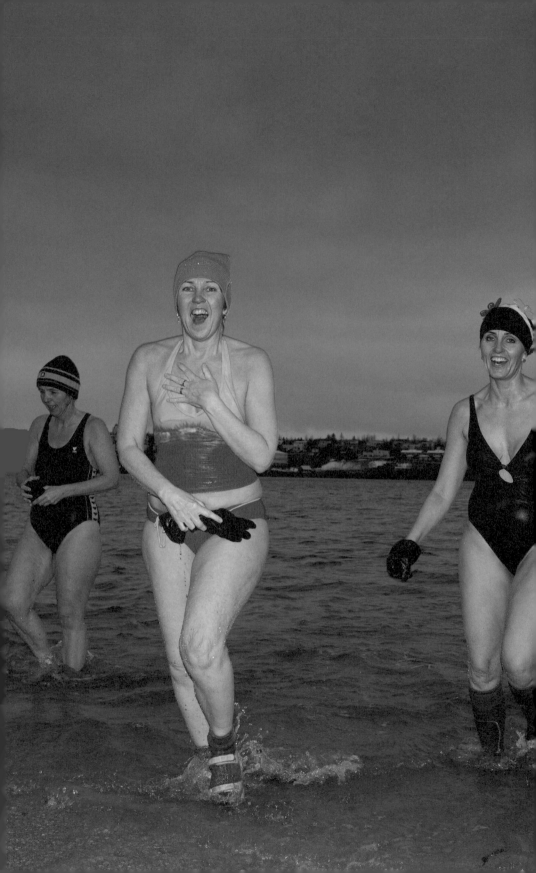

WINTER SWIMMING LINGO

- Shield-maiden, pirate, Viking – a winter swimmer.

- Baptism by fire – the first plunge into the cold water, often combined with a ceremony or celebration.

- Radiator swimmer, or dry swimmer – someone who has a sauna before their first plunge.

- Dopamine-lover – winter swimmers who can be in the water for a long time, or just love to cold-water swim.

- Champagne under the skin – the bubbling/prickling feeling in your skin when you go into the water a second time, or get out of the water again.

- Eyes at eye level – it's a saying about looking each other in the eye, and not at each other's naked bodies.

- Keep right on the steps – you say this to remind people to share space on the steps and not cluster on the jetty.

- Saunagus – aromatherapy in the sauna. A "saunagus master" pours water and essential oils on the hot stones. This evaporates into a fragrant, oil-infused steam, which is distributed throughout the sauna with a large fan or towel.

Opposite: "Champagne under the skin", Nauthólsvík, Reykjavik, Iceland.

CHAPTER 9

DANGER AND SAFETY IN COLD WATER

"Swimming is a confusing sport, because
sometimes you do it for fun, and other
times you do it to not die!"

DEMETRI MARTIN
Comedian and author

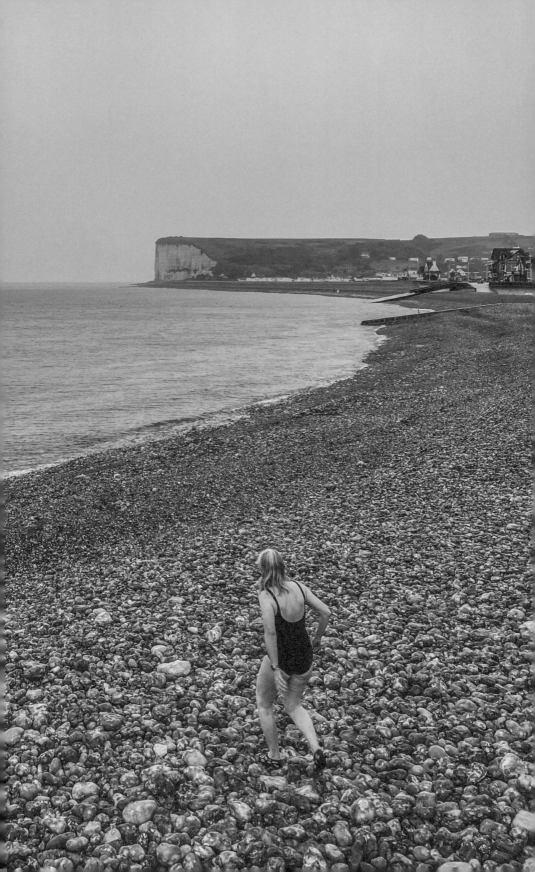

*To allay your concerns (if you have any), let's start
with the conclusion: winter swimming is safe if you
take precautions. "How can that be?" you may wonder.
Allow me to share some exciting research into human
physiological responses to cold water, and hopefully
answer questions such as: What temperature defines
cold water? What are the signs of hypothermia?
Why are people with heart disease at risk? And, can
habituation increase our chances of survival? I hope
this chapter will help you feel safe and informed on
your winter swimming journey.*

The statistics

Drowning in water, hot or cold, is the third most common cause of
accidental death in the world, accounting for 7 per cent of all injury-
related deaths. The World Health Organization (WHO) estimates
that in 2015, 360,000 people (forty per hour) died by drowning.
WHO believes that the number of deaths is underestimated due
to poor reporting in many developing countries. Because drowning
is so common worldwide, and because of the prominence of tragic

drowning accidents in history, such as the sinking of the *Titanic*, it is more common for research to focus on cold water as a "killer" than as a cure for diseases.

A study from 2014 reported 1,094 cases of drowning or near drowning in open water in the USA between 1975 and 1996. Most cases (78 per cent) had bad outcomes (74 per cent resulted in death, 4 per cent in severe neurological consequences), and of those with good outcomes, 88 per cent were submerged for less than six minutes in cold water (and survived with no neurological consequences). The researchers found that submersion time was the most powerful predictor of a good (alive) or bad outcome (death), and that there was a very low likelihood of a good outcome if submersion exceeded ten minutes. But what about the impact of the cold water temperatures?

The researchers reviewed the scientific literature on survival in cold temperatures and found low temperature to be protective. They concluded that if water temperature is warmer than 6°C (43°F), survival/resuscitation is extremely unlikely if submerged longer than thirty minutes. If water temperature is 6°C or below, survival/resuscitation is extremely unlikely if submerged longer than ninety minutes. It may seem a little contradictory that the chances of survival are higher with colder temperatures even below 6°C. The explanation is that cooling slows down the processes in the brain and body, thereby avoiding hypoxic brain damage. It seems, therefore, that the likelihood of survival depends on both colder temperatures and, not surprisingly, the duration of submersion.

Cold water - a broad concept

Cold water activates the sympathetic nervous system, i.e. the cold-shock response, which prepares you to survive what could be a life-threatening situation. The body perceives being in water of less than 15°C (59°F) as a threat, especially if you're in for more than

Page 154: Going for it on the Opal coast, Normandy, France.

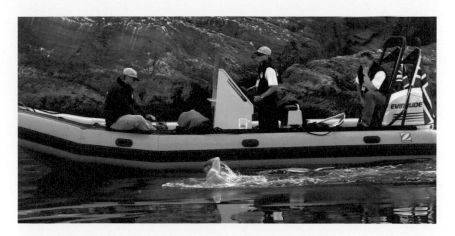

Above: Lewis Gordon Pugh swims around the plateau of Nordkapp, Norway.

thirty minutes. But winter swimming as a sport is a voluntary and controlled activity, and the risk of accidents is reduced when you take precautions.

Water freezes at different temperatures. As seawater freezes at -1.9°C (28.5°F), and human tissue at -0.55°C (33°F), it is possible to get frostbite when winter swimming, though it rarely happens. Caution is advised when swimming in pools and in seas near the Polar Regions in winter. The salt in the sea and chlorine added to the water in swimming pools enable the water to remain liquid at sub-zero temperatures, and swimming in such waters is much more challenging and dangerous. An example was featured in the *Telegraph* in 2012, where Lewis Gordon Pugh, an experienced ice swimmer, swam near the North Pole in -1.7°C (28.9°F). He suffered frostbite in his fingers and it took him four months to regain the feeling in his hands.

Winter swimming can feel colder at certain times than at others, even if the water temperature is the same. This is partly due to environmental factors that influence our perception of the cold, such as currents in the water and wind speed (which will increase or lower the wind-chill factor). The wind-chill factor is the actual cooling in temperature when the wind blows heat away from bare skin, in relation to the air temperature measured with a thermometer. Note the air temperature and wind speed per hour and you can easily work out the wind-chill factor using a calculator. The effect of wet skin is not taken into account in this calculation, but it's certainly a factor that contributes to the feeling of cold: chill factor X wet skin = freezing cold! Let's call it "the winter swimmer equation". Wind and water temperature alone are probably too limited to be able to constitute the definition of "cold water" when swimming.

> A neutral water temperature for a naked person at rest is about 35°C (95°F). If the person remains in the water the body will lose heat, the core temperature will decrease and eventually they will get cold.

Hypothermia

As the body cools, it gradually shuts down vital bodily functions. Untrained winter swimmers can retain mobility for between ten and thirteen minutes in water below 5°C (41°F). At these low temperatures, it is only cold-habituated and trained ice swimmers who can stay in the water for longer. Being in the water for longer than thirty minutes can lead to hypothermia, i.e. having a core body temperature of less than 35°C (95°F), which can cause vascular and nerve damage and lead to serious injury or even death. The definition of hypothermia came in the wake of the *Titanic* disaster and was later confirmed with information gathered from battles on the high seas during World War II. But there is no similarly precise definition of "cold water". Given that some unpleasant reactions to cold water can occur between 10°C and 15°C (50°F and 60°F), it is probably fair to say that "cold water" is water at or below 15°C.

Symptoms of hypothermia

As soon as you get into cold water the body begins to cool down. In the initial stages of the cooling process, you feel cold, pain and tingling in the skin, then a stinging in fingers and toes which moves to other parts of the body such as thighs, abdomen and back. At this stage you're not close to hypothermia. In unhabituated winter swimmers, the initial cold pain will last from twenty seconds to a minute, at which point the cold numbs the skin and hyperventilation decreases. To protect against the high heat loss to the water, the body increases the metabolism by activating brown fat and skeletal muscles. You will feel this as slight shivering. When the shivering starts it's time to get out of the water before the next stage of the cooling process occurs, when everything begins to move slower. It feels as though your skin is tightening, your muscles become stiff and you can't move. At this stage the head feels cold at first, then a tingling and stinging

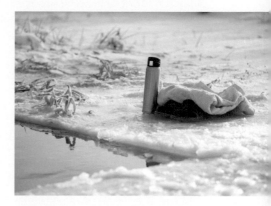

A hot drink on standby is a good idea.

sets in, before a kind of paralysis combined with "brain freeze". Your breathing is also affected and slows, and speech becomes difficult. The condition is evident both visibly and audibly either in yourself or in others. The body is struggling to maintain its temperature at this point and you're not well. You could go into convulsions.

It is, of course, advisable to act before these symptoms occur. Get out of the water – put a bathrobe or dryrobe on – put your hands in your armpits – go somewhere warm! Lie down if you feel dizzy, or lean forward and get your head below heart level until you feel the dizziness subside. Consumption of alcohol before swimming in very cold water should be avoided, as this will accelerate the onset and progression of hypothermia.

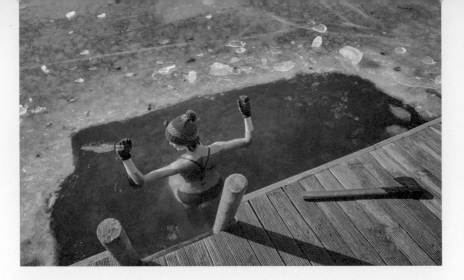

Above: Wearing a neoprene hat or beanie minimizes heat loss from the head. Holding hands above the water also protects against hypothermia.

As mentioned earlier, the cold shock also causes a 30 per cent decrease in blood flow to the brain. This may result in dizziness, which increases the risk of drowning in the event that you lose consciousness in the water. The low blood supply to the brain is obviously one of the main reasons why swimming alone is not advised. Nor is submerging your head in cold water. In general, we lose 80 per cent of our body heat via the head. The head is bare, highly vascularized and has a high surface area. The veins in the head, unlike those in the rest of the body, do not have the same capacity to contract and dilate when exposed to cold and hot temperatures. So when the head is submerged in cold water the cold-shock response increases dramatically, along with the rate of heat loss and the risk of hypothermia. Have you ever wondered why winter swimmers wear a beanie or bobble hat in the water? It's simple – the beanie minimizes heat loss from the head and keeps you warmer for longer. A neoprene hat is also a good addition to your kit if you submerge your head when swimming.

It is generally believed that the risk of hypothermia and drowning, even in icy water, does not occur until you've been in cold water for at least fifteen minutes. Hypothermia affects all the cells in the body and their ability to function optimally. If you go into hypothermia, the

Symptoms of hypothermia as core temperature decreases in cold water:

- 36°C (96.8°F) – the body begins to shiver visibly, the heart rate increases and breathing is affected. This is usually the point people know to get out of the water and seek warmth, if not before. If you didn't know – this is your heads up!

- 35°C (95°F) – confusion and disorientation; diminished muscle coordination.

- 34°C (93°F) – memory loss.

- 33°C (91°F) – onset of cardiac arrhythmia.

- 33–30°C (91–86°F) – consciousness gradually reduced; rigid muscle tone, shivering stops.

- 30°C (86°F) – loss of consciousness, hypotension and low respiration.

- 28°C (82°F) – heart fibrillation and barely any respiration.

- 25°C (77°F) – cardiac arrest and death.

body's cells can no longer perform: blood flow and nerve functions are affected, and this becomes evident in the various ways described above. Knowing the sequence of symptoms associated with slowly decreasing body temperature will, hopefully, make you aware and able to react in time.

There are some variations between the body's core temperature and symptoms of hypothermia, but 25°C (77°F) is the body temperature most often associated with death from hypothermia.

Still, there have been survivors with even lower body temperatures. Incredibly, a child of twenty-seven months had the lowest-recorded core body temperature ever observed at 11.8°C (53.2°F) after accidental exposure to cold. The coldest adult survivor had a core body temperature of 13.7°C (56.6°F) degrees after being in very cold water.

There is also variation in the speed at which people reach hypothermia. The factors are a combination of different environmental conditions such as air and water temperature, and water movement and current, as already mentioned. There are other factors relating to the individual, such as body insulation – i.e. the amount of white fat – body size, muscle mass, blood sugar and sex. Some of these are explained in the following sections.

Survival and cold habituation

The effects of cold water range from beneficial to harmful depending on the close interplay between the different factors mentioned above, including time spent in the water. Other important factors are the degree of cold habituation and the body's composition of fat and muscle. Fat and muscle mass play a role in insulation and heat production, and therefore determine how long you can stay in the water before becoming hypothermic. Several studies have shown that overweight people who are acclimatized are more likely to tolerate a longer stay in cold water compared to people of average weight who are not acclimatized. Interestingly, a study from 2015 shows that an overweight ice swimmer with a BMI over 35 kg/m² and approximately 45 per cent body fat never became hypothermic, even after several sessions in ice-cold water. Even more fascinating is a case report from 1986 which describes an Icelandic fisherman who survived in ice-cold water, probably due to his high proportion of adipose tissue. The boat

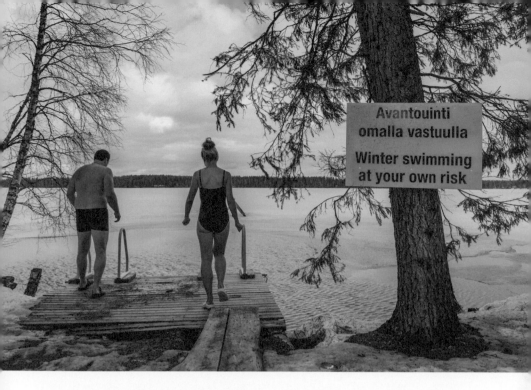

Above: "At their own risk", Lapland, Finland.

---

sank and two other fishermen drowned within ten minutes, whereas he swam back to shore in 5°C (41°F) sea – an ordeal which took him approximately six hours to complete.

Other scientific studies have shown the beneficial effects of spending protracted periods in the water if one is habituated to the cold, and that the core temperature in cold-habituated subjects with normal BMI decreased just as fast as in non-habituated subjects with the same BMI (between 18.5 to 24.9) when sitting still in cold water. Therefore, the increased chance of survival is probably not solely attributed to temperature-protecting characteristics, such as the amount of white fat. Instead, it might be the improved ability to use muscles to move in cold water – and to panic less – which increases the chances of survival. This was shown in a study from 1995, in which nine men wearing survival suits were immersed in 3.6°C (38.5°F) water. It was discovered that periods of movement gave a better chance of survival compared to continuous heat production by muscle shivering alone.

When you're in direct contact with cold water, there is a difference between convective and conductive water flow. Convective heat loss is the transfer of heat from a body to moving molecules such as air or liquid. Heat loss can occur by conduction of heat from the skin to the cold water around the body. It has been shown that heat loss is greater in wind and waves. However, if muscles are moving at the same time, by swimming, heat production is increased, and with it the chance of survival.

Habituation and performance depends on cold-water training, the weather and our physiology – and not only on willpower. Body composition should be taken into account when comparing one ice swimmer with another, and competitions should perhaps be organized into different weight classes.

Avoid winter swimming if you suffer from:

- Untreated coronary artery disease and/or chest pain (angina pectoris).

- Untreated high blood pressure.

- Severe heart rhythm disturbances.

(Recommendations by the Danish Heart Association)

Cold-water swimming and cardiac risk

Swimming in cold water is a significant cause of death globally, but it is worth remembering that deaths most typically occur as the result of an accident. If you are generally in good health, it should be safe for you to become a winter swimmer.

Recent scientific studies have suggested that a large proportion of cold-water immersion deaths can be attributed to arrhythmia resulting from activation of the sympathetic and parasympathetic nervous system, also called the "autonomic conflict". In some people

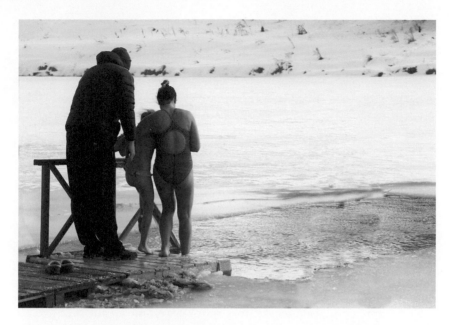

Above: Children should be under constant supervision when in cold water.

with pre-existing conditions, the reactive autonomic response may provoke arrhythmia and result in cardiac arrest. As explained in Chapter 5 (The Cold-Shock Response), receptors located in the skin react to cold water and activate the sympathetic nervous system (cold shock). If waves splash into your face, this will cause increased vagal stimulation and diving response. This autonomic conflict probably plays a crucial role in triggering dysrhythmias and arrhythmias in the heart. Importantly, studies show that for fatal arrhythmias to occur during cold-water immersion, predisposing factors such as Long QT syndrome, coronary artery disease or myocardial hypertrophy must be present. But non-fatal arrhythmias can still result in death indirectly if a healthy person becomes hypothermic to the extent that they lose muscle coordination, and they breathe in water and drown as a result. Drowning leads to cardiac arrest within two minutes. So even if you're healthy, stay safe by going carefully into the water holding on to a ladder or rope. If it's a day with high waves, consider postponing your swim to a less windy day.

The purpose of cold habituation is to protect the body from hypothermia by improving heat production, metabolism, insulation and blood circulation. Luckily it's this physiological protection of your body temperature which brings health benefits. Tricking the body into reacting as if you're going to die is certainly a bold way of keeping healthy! In fact, randomly shocking the body may bring it closer to the environments of our early Stone Age ancestors. And yet, unlike the sudden appearance of a bear, winter swimming is (if precautions are taken) predictable, controlled, safe and a very exciting activity to add to your health mission.

Children and winter swimming

More and more children are now practising winter swimming with their parents or grandparents. It is particularly important that adults are attuned to the safety of their children, and educate them as to the signals their bodies send them. If they experience the cold-shock response, they should be reassured if they begin to hyperventilate. It's easy to panic if you don't feel prepared. Compared to adults, children typically have a higher body surface area-to-body mass ratio and less body fat. A research study from 1973 shows that this leads to a greater decrease in core temperature in children (at 20°C/68°F). Another study from 1992 shows that eleven- to twelve-year-old boys with the same amount of body-fat percentage as adult men between nineteen and thity-four years maintained the same core temperature in an air temperature of 5°C (41°F), both at rest and during exercise. The mechanism for achieving this was different, however. During cooling, the boys' blood vessels had a better capacity to contract, resulting in lower skin temperature. They achieved a higher energy burn than the men, probably as a result of muscle shivering. Overall, this shows that children get cold faster than adults, but that they compensate for a drop in core temperature by increasing energy metabolism. They use the energy in their muscles, and will therefore tire more quickly in the cold than adults. Because of this, it is advised that children should

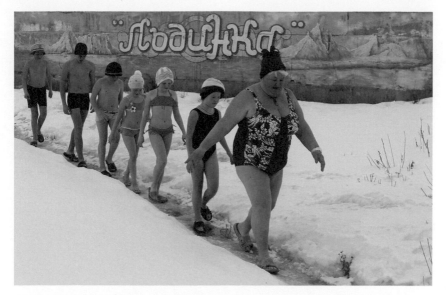

Above: Zinaida Bulygina, former winter marathon champion swimmer, leads young members of the *Ldinka* (Ice Floe) club to the icy waters of the Tuba river at Kuragino, Siberia, Russia.

be under constant supervision when in cold water. And for safety reasons, children should avoid swimming in water below 15°C (59°F), but simply take a quick dip for a few seconds and then get back into the warmth right away.

The afterdrop

The first time I went into very cold water, I immersed myself for only a few seconds. I used to be one of those people who was always cold. So I made quite a scene on the steps when I started hyperventilating, even before I'd dipped a toe in. It's years ago now, but I will always remember the overwhelming feeling of the cold wind and the ice under my feet. My whole body was screaming GET OUT OF THIS! Panic is the right word. Today the experience is very different, as I have developed a method for enduring the cold using nasal breathing and mindfulness to stay calm through the short-term stress. But back then I was challenged. I had barely touched the water before I felt panic throughout my body, and when I got home I lay shivering under a blanket on the sofa. When I started reading up about it, I found it was common after cold-water swimming – it's called "the afterdrop".

The physiological explanation

Afterdrop is the phenomenon of your body temperature continuing to fall after you get out of cold water. The drop in core temperature can continue for forty or even sixty minutes after you exit the water. When you swim in cold water the body activates the flight-or-fight response, where the blood is directed to the inner organs through peripheral vasoconstriction. This process helps you stay in the water longer. Shortly after you exit the water, peripheral vasoconstriction ends, but the cooling process does not stop straightaway. Cold blood from your limbs and skin returns to the core, where it mixes with warmer blood. This causes your core body temperature to drop, even if you're warmly dressed and move into a warm environment. The cold layer of skin and muscles continues to cool the core, bringing on shivering or feeling faint and unwell, and potentially hypothermia. The cooling process (afterdrop) is caused by "conductive cooling" and vasodilation as blood returns to the skin.

Warm up naturally

In one of my studies we trained unhabituated participants to become winter swimmers. One of the participants was still nervous about getting cold, and it was her first week in the experiment. We met with her on the jetty and talked through the method before she took a quick dip and headed for the sauna. An hour later I got a text from her: "Hi Susanna, I just got home. You always advise us to keep moving when we get home, to increase thermogenesis, and I did! But I'm still literally shivering my ass off on my sofa!"

Even though she had kept moving to keep her muscles warm, she did eventually feel the afterdrop when she sat down. After following my participants during this initial stage of the study, I found that the

Breathing: a guide

Just before you step into the water, exhale through your mouth, so your lungs are empty of air. When you've exhaled completely, put your first foot in – taking long breaths in through your nose and exhaling deeply through your mouth – and walk decisively down the steps until the water is at your shoulders. As you're going in, continue to focus on breathing calmly and deeply. Think about relaxing and count "one, two, three . . ." for up to twenty seconds. After this point it becomes easier to breathe and stay calm.

afterdrop is much more profound in new winter swimmers. Once habituation is built up, the body becomes much more efficient at rewarming by activating the brown fat and skeletal muscles.

Minimizing the afterdrop

So, the key to minimizing the afterdrop and staying well is to warm up slowly and gradually. My experience and advice is to keep moving your muscles after your swim. Get dressed quickly and warmly. You may feel fantastic immediately after swimming as the cooled blood has not yet returned to your core. Best to wrap up warm before it does. Once you're dressed, start moving your body: power walk, do the horse stance or some star jumps, dance around, cycle home, clean the house etc. . . . The point is to let your body reheat naturally but slowly. If you go straight home and take a hot shower, you'll probably start to shiver and feel colder. It will increase vasodilation in the skin, the blood will be cooled, which will increase the rate at which cooled blood returns to the core and makes the afterdrop faster and deeper. Instead, wait until you've warmed up again. Drink something hot.

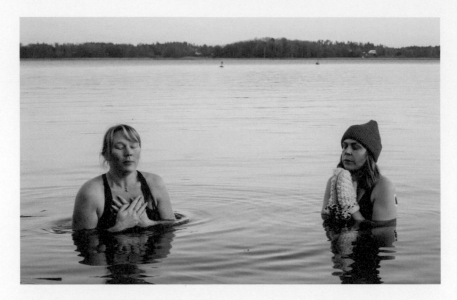

Above: Just breathe – Norrtälje, Stockholm County, Sweden.

Shivering is very energy consuming, which may be good for increasing metabolism, but keep the shivering to a minimum and don't make it your goal. You know your body best – don't compete with others, and bear in mind that you'll continue to get colder after swimming. Adjust your time in the water according to your own adaptation, and to the weather and temperature conditions.

Afterdrop and habituation

Before I started my studies I experimented with not taking a hot shower after a cold swim. I found that reheating naturally was the safest and most efficient method. Within a few months my body was reheating so fast that I begin to feel warm again as soon as I got home. Was I still cold? Slightly, yes, but the activation of my brown fat and muscles was swift, and the shivering was at a minimum.

But what if you don't shiver? Wouldn't that decrease the core temperature still further? Here is my take on this: habituation and the lack of major muscle shivering is not a sign of the body being less capable of protecting the core temperature. In fact it's the opposite.

Brown fat and muscle cells have become more mitochondria-rich, and more efficient at heat generation. This minimizes shivering, which then becomes less obvious to the eye. If you measure the core temperature of habituated and unhabituated cold-water swimmers, the habituated swimmers protect their core temperature just as well, but with less shivering. This is probably due to increased thermogenesis and metabolism.

Hang in there for three sessions

Several times a week for my research we met with untrained winter swimmers to guide and motivate their training. One morning, one of the women was going into the water for the first time. She was excited and happy to be part of a winter swimming club and she'd been wanting to winter swim for many years. Now it was finally happening! We were going to follow the usual course of action – go out to the jetty, down into the water, breathe calmly (or at least try to), get out again, wrap up in a towel and go to the sauna.

"I want to do this, but I'm just so nervous," she said, apologetically.

"That's understandable," I said, to calm her. "But it's a quick dip and you'll make it. Just get out of the water when you've had enough."

We went out on the jetty. There was no wind, but the air was cold. The sun was peeking out from behind the white clouds. The water temperature read 10°C (50°F), and the air temperature 11°C (52°F). A beautiful October day, we agreed, and perfect for a first plunge. On the jetty we went over the process again. Now she felt ready! She went resolutely down the steps and continued at the same pace into the water until it reached her shoulders. It went as expected; as soon as she hit the water, she started gasping and hyperventilating, clearly the cold-shock response had been activated. She got out of the water and the other swimmers praised her for her first dip. She was laughing. It was great! You could tell that she was happy and very proud. We went to the sauna and took two more dips, alternating with sauna sessions. She was excited and the "winter swimmer's high" was very

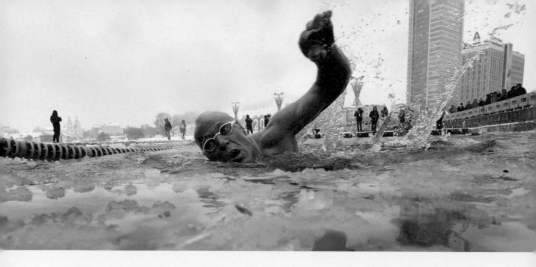

Above: A participant in the Minsk Open winter swimming championship in the Svisloch river near Minsk Sports Palace, Belarus.

---

evident. However, between the three dips she also complained that the shortness of breath was uncomfortable. We performed breathing exercises with her, which helped a lot. But then the next day she called and confessed that she was insecure about the whole winter swimming idea.

"It's cold and I felt my body react really strongly! I didn't feel like I could get any air! I'm not sure that I can do winter swimming," she said.

She was clearly stressed and panicking, thinking back on her first session, although she'd handled it as expected for a first plunge. Many people find the experience challenging and it sometimes takes a lot of courage to do it again. We talked and praised her for challenging herself. One shouldn't expect the full Zen feeling right at the beginning, as the body is unhabituated to the cold water and nerves often take over. This is all very normal, as is feeling a shortness of breath. The overwhelming feeling will be there the first few times, but the body learns fast and one will quickly notice the difference. So hang in there! Luckily, this nervous swimmer decided not to give up, and the research team and I met with her again so she'd have support. After another three or four trips into the water she had completely changed the way she felt about winter swimming.

"It's a lot better now – I can control my breathing better and enjoy the plunges more and more. Now I just need to keep going!" she said. She was a much calmer – though still new – winter swimmer, and she kept it up for the rest of the season. It was wonderful to see. She was proud of herself and felt empowered by the challenge. What a triumph for her!

Having the support of other winter swimmers will keep you motivated and safe. It is often decisive in determining whether cold-water swimming will get "under your skin". Winter swimmers often say that once you've reached this point in your training, you won't want to do without. As a habituated winter swimmer myself, I couldn't agree more.

Breathing

Shortness of breath and muscle fatigue are challenges in many forms of sport. It takes time for the body to adapt physically to new surroundings and demands, so think of it as a journey and relax. The main strategy for reducing shortness of breath is to avoid panicking by breathing calmly and deeply as you enter the water. A breathing technique gives you something concrete to focus on, which in itself can foster calmness and help you to increase your time in the icy water.

Even if your brain is shouting "HELP!" and your breathing is out of rhythm, know that you will get it right after a few times. When you do, it will completely change your winter swimming or dipping experience. Doing the deep exhalation before hitting cold water gives your lungs greater capacity to breathe in more air, more deeply. This way you avoid shallow breathing, panic and the risk of drowning. By the time you've been in the cold water three times you'll have suddenly mastered this, and other people will wonder how you did it. Please share tips on how to breathe while winter swimming, and thereby increase general safety.

COLD FACTS: HOW TO SWIM SAFELY IN COLD WATER

- You must be able to swim before attempting to swim in very cold water.

- Avoid winter swimming if you suffer from: untreated coronary artery disease and/or chest pain (angina pectoris), untreated high blood pressure or severe heart rhythm disturbances. If in doubt, consult your GP.

- It is advised that children should take only a quick dip, and they must be under the supervision of adults at all times.

- Never swim alone – make sure you have a swimming buddy at your side.

- Never swim in open water if you are under the influence of alcohol or feel unwell.

- Take a first aid course – you'll know how to respond in case of an emergency.

- Find out where the defibrillator is in your winter swimming club.

- Pay attention to where a lifebuoy is located.

- Always carry a charged phone so you can call for help – consider putting your phone in a waterproof container.

- Consider using a swimming buoy or flotation device.

- Wear a swimming cap, goggles and headlamp if you plan to swim in the dark hours of winter.

- Avoid dunking your head into cold water, as this increases the autonomic conflict and accelerates heat loss.

- Wear a neoprene hat or beanie to keep your head warm and to slow or minimize heat loss.

- Walk slowly on docks, jetties and steps as they may be slippery due to ice or moss. Wearing neoprene shoes makes it safer to walk and less cold.

- Breathe deeply and calmly as you get into the water, to minimize hyperventilation.

- Take a short dip the first time you winter swim, for example, one to ten seconds. Then you can increase the length of your plunges as habituation increases and you have better control of your breathing.

- Put on warm clothes after swimming and drink a hot beverage. Warm up naturally by moving your body.

- Be aware of undercurrents as you go into the water.

- Try to remove ice before you get into the water. Ice chunks can be sharp, and there is a risk you may cut yourself. If you do, you're unlikely to notice, as the cold water numbs the nerves in the skin.

- Never swim beneath ice – there is a risk of panic and drowning.

CHAPTER 10

DOES IT MAKE YOU HEALTHIER?

"What doesn't kill you makes you stronger"

NIETZSCHE
Philosopher

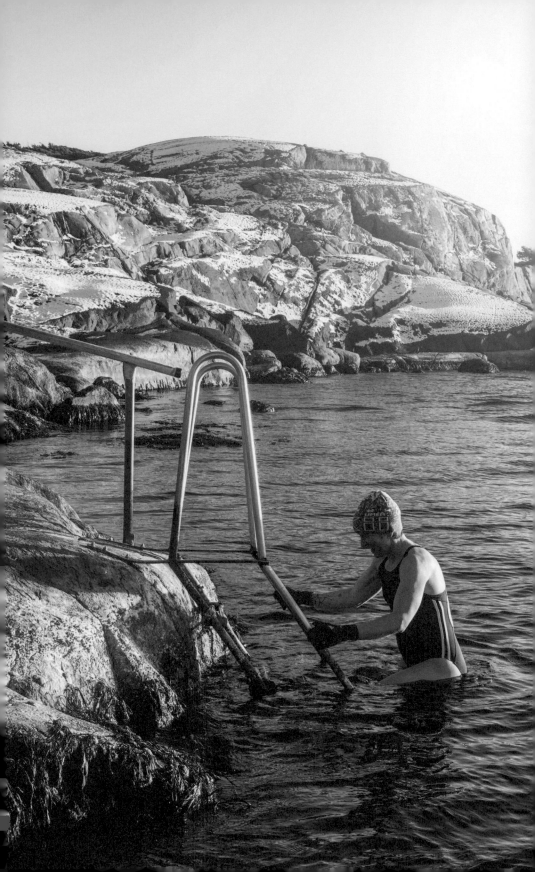

10

Everyone needs to exercise to stay healthy – that's no surprise. The question is whether winter swimming is in fact exercise? The short answer is, yes! You are exercising, even just by getting out of the house and preparing for your swim. But that's not the main reason. Cold-water immersion is a special form of endurance sport. In this chapter we will dive into the science around the physiological health benefits and explain how and why cold water is exercise.

If you ask me, it's a little investment with a rather big health contribution. Several studies have suggested that cold-water swimming has a wide variety of health benefits, not only for general well-being, but also for the amelioration of mood disorders, changes in insulin sensitivity, hematological and endocrine function, and a reduction in upper respiratory tract infections. These benefits are outlined in this chapter, and I'm going to go into a bit of scientific detail to explain them.

In general, swimming is good cardio training, with health benefits that can help to prevent major lifestyle diseases such as heart disease, cardiovascular diseases and diabetes. The cold water that surrounds your body is associated with significant physiological changes that may

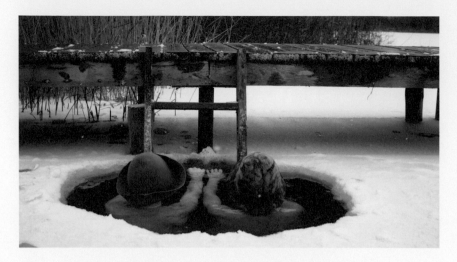

Above: A felt hat reduces heat loss in cold water, and protects your head from the heat in the sauna.

Page 178: It helps to keep smiling.

be particularly beneficial, due to an increased tolerance for cold and a cascade of neurotransmitters and hormones. Is it possible to feel the health benefits? This will depend on the overall state of your health. If you have joint pain, studies show that people may immediately feel pain relief in cold water. Apart from this, most of the beneficial effects are measurable, though not necessarily evident as something you directly feel or sense. The body has to be able to cope with a significant stress response, so if you suffer from heart problems, it is essential to be cautious when starting out. If you suffer from joint pain, atherosclerosis, stress, low energy or mood swings, it has been shown that there are particular health benefits to be gained from cold water. If you are not affected by any of these conditions, it is still beneficial in a preventive way – and of course it's better to prevent a disease than to treat one.

A global questionnaire responded to by more than eight hundred winter swimmers and sauna users shows that the positive impact of cold water on mood and energy is universal, and independent of any health conditions. On the more anecdotal side, I often listen to winter swimming stories from people all over the world which describe the impact of enhanced mood and energy on their quality of life, and the event is often described as life changing. These accounts are fascinating and inspiring, and confirm that there is much more research that could be done to understand the effects of cold-water swimming. For me, hearing these stories makes all the scientific studies and evidence come alive.

Brown fat and sleep

Conditions that affect your health and winter swimming outcomes are chronic stress and a lack of sleep. Sleep is very important to our metabolism. If the circadian rhythm is out of balance, it disrupts precisely those hormones (e.g. leptin, cortisol and serotonin) that are known to regulate basic functions such as hunger and sleep. It's a malevolent cycle: too little or disrupted sleep affects signals sent from the intestines and liver to the satiety centre in the brain, where it disturbs what you feel like eating, and when. So a lack of sleep can lead to poor eating habits with excess caloric intake, which in turn can make you tired.

You'll get the best outcomes from exercise, including winter swimming, if you are not stressed and/or tired. Too much to ask for? Of course, as we cannot always be in the perfect healthy balance, but it's possible that winter swimming can positively affect this balance and sleep quality. Anecdotally, winter swimmers often claim to sleep better. In line with this, research studies show that cold water decreases inflammation and could be a way of treating joint pain and mood disorders, which are conditions that impact sleep quality. From a broader perspective, a 2015 scientific report shows that sleep disturbances correlate with obesity and other metabolic diseases.

An important regulator of cortisol levels in our body is a protein called IL-6, which appears to play a significant role in conditions related to chronic stress and aging. A clinical trial from 2000 shows that high IL-6 levels in the blood during sleep are associated with bad sleep quality (which has been shown in people with depression) and with a risk of inflammatory disease. Could IL-6 be regulated by winter swimming? We don't yet know the answer to this. Another parameter regulated by stressors such as cold is the brown fat, as discussed in Chapter 7 (Brown Fat).

More recent studies from 2015 to 2020 show that activation of brown fat increases metabolic rate. They also show that repeated cooling with air or using a pharmacological treatment called Mirabegron causes sympathetic activation and increases insulin sensitivity and brown fat activity. Given the above-mentioned metabolic benefits, an improved regulation of brown fat in humans could be a potential strategy to counteract the development of metabolic diseases. We also know that immersion in cold water results in sympathetic activation, so does this activation also apply to winter swimming? We know that swimming in cold water for just one minute or less increases noradrenalin blood levels two- to four-fold. This was shown in a study from 2001, which also demonstrates that regularly practised winter swimming attenuates this increase, due to cold adaptation. The mechanism is not quite understood. But as noradrenalin activates the cells in the body and that process increases mitochondria in the cells, it may be that less noradrenalin is needed the more mitochondria there are. More mitochondria means that the cells in, for example, brown fat will activate faster and generate heat with less noradrenalin – like a well-oiled machine. This means that, in theory, the cold water should activate brown fat as soon as we go into the water, but also that the body adapts. It is possible that the adaptation is related to the increased activation of brown fat that occurs during cold acclimatization, although this has not yet been explored in winter swimmers.

In my research, therefore, we hypothesized that winter swimmers would have a different brown fat activation – perhaps more active when exposed to cold, or a greater proportion of brown fat – compared to a healthy control group. It seems that the regulators of sleep and

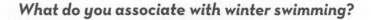

What do you associate with winter swimming?

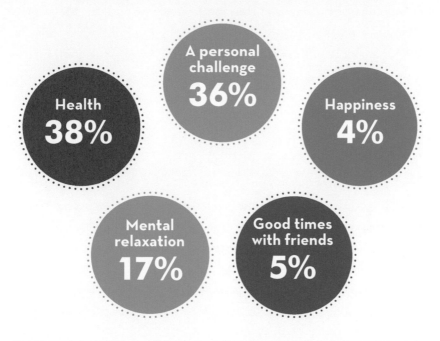

From the author's questionnaire of non-winter swimmers.

metabolism might be connected. It would be interesting to measure levels of cortisol, IL-6, leptin and brown fat for a day and night in winter swimmers compared to a control group, in order to potentially establish a different sleeping pattern in winter swimmers. As you've probably guessed, these were some of the outcomes from my PhD studies in brown fat and diurnal rhythm in winter swimmers. If the parameters are different in winter swimmers, cold-water swimming might be a gateway (read "small-time investment") to better sleep and an improved health balance.

Activating the immune system
New winter swimmers often dread their first dip because they are nervous about their physiological reactions to the cold water.

Most people focus on questions such as: What happens when I hit the cold water? Will I be able to breathe? What if I panic? After the immediate issues of survival have been dealt with, most new winter swimmers are preoccupied with the risk of getting ill. "Am I going to be ill for a couple of days now?" many people ask. In my experience it rarely happens. Most people who become ill after a cold-water dip will have already caught a virus before their swim. As an example, a new winter swimmer from my experiments caught a cold shortly after his first dip. Why would this have happened? It's all to do with balance in the immune system.

Icy water triggers the immune system, and probably protects it from respiratory diseases in the upper part of the lungs. In fact, a major study from 1999 has shown that the incidence of upper respiratory tract infections such as colds, sinusitis and sore throats decreased by 40 per cent in experienced winter swimmers, due to improved antioxidant protection. A 2015 study investigated the incidence and severity of upper airway infections in fifty cold-water swimmers and their partners (non-swimmers and indoor pool swimmers). Cold-water swimmers reported significantly fewer respiratory tract infections. Surprisingly, though, the authors found no differences in the effect of wild winter swimming and pool winter swimming on the immune system.

On the anecdotal side, winter swimmers claim they feel healthier and have fewer sick days than before they took up the activity. They experience a significant decrease in the number of infections, having them less frequently and more mildly, and some go several years without colds or other illness. However, scientific data on sick days and winter swimmers are mostly retrospective, which increases the risk of "recall-bias"; that is, not being able to remember the number of sick days in the past. It is more accurate to measure forwards and track winter swimmers reporting events as they occur. An example of such is a clinical trial on cold showers, mentioned earlier, which measured sick days for a period of ninety days. Researchers found that taking

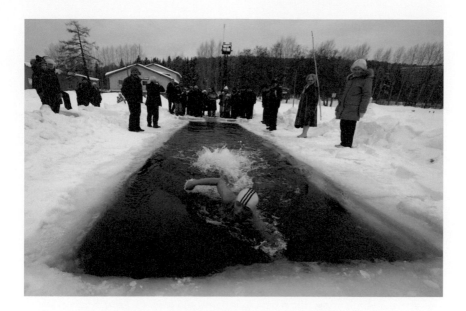

Above: A winter swimmimg competitor at the Verkh-Neyvinsky pond near the town of Novouralsk in the Ural Mountains, Russia.

cold showers for thirty seconds for thirty days decreased sick leave from work. The results are interesting and suggest that the immune system is positively influenced in the health of winter swimmers. But are there any plausible biological explanations for these observations?

Studies from 1977 and 1989 report that cold water gives immediate pain relief for rheumatoid arthritis and muscle ache, and can increase joint mobility. They suggest that these benefits can be explained by an improved immune system due to the release of stress hormones such as noradrenalin triggered by cold exposure. Also, experienced winter swimmers have been found to have higher levels of white blood cells (leucocytes and monocytes) as compared to control groups. This was evident in a study from 2011 of ice swimmers before and after a 150-metre (164-yard) winter swim at 6°C (43°F), from which authors concluded that greater protection against inflammation and respiratory infections is very likely. It suggests an improvement in the body's response to stress.

Monocytes are the body's "waste-disposal team" and have the task of eradicating and absorbing foreign organisms – e.g. viruses and inflammation in the blood vessels. Scientists have looked into this closely and compared winter swimmers and non-winter swimmers. They found higher levels of interleukins-1-beta and 6, which are proteins that help to strengthen the immune system in winter swimmers. It was also found that interleukins-1-beta and 6 decreased in untrained winter swimmers getting into cold water, while an increase was measured in experienced winter swimmers. This suggests that the acclimatizing mechanisms of regular winter swimming may strengthen the immune system.

So, a cold-water dip by an untrained winter swimmer is more stressful to the body, and the immune system can take a short-lived nosedive, which may allow for a potential virus to take over. Maybe you remember catching a cold after a particularly stressful period? This is due to a dip in the immune system. Chronic stress is bad for you and you don't adapt, whereas short-term stress from cold water hardens your immune system. For new winter swimmers, my advice is to choose a day to start when you feel unstressed and well. With increased habituation, you will boost your immune system and improve antioxidant protection.

Improved antioxidant protection

The immune system works via several mechanisms and also comprises an antioxidant system which protects against free radicals. The free radicals are atoms that are eager to interact with other elements, because they themselves lack an electron – so they sneak up on other cells to steal one! Then the other molecule will lack an electron and therefore becomes a new free radical – and so it goes on. This chain reaction can cause major damage to cell walls, proteins, neurotransmitters and all other cells in the body.

We cannot avoid free radicals. They are found in processed foods, alcohol, tobacco smoke, pesticides, air pollutants and more.

Free radicals come from oxidative stress, and when a free radical steals an electron, the process is called "oxidation". Oxidative stress is a disturbance in the balance between free radicals and antioxidants. Antioxidants, on the other hand, deliver an electron to the free radicals without becoming a free radical themselves, as they are repaired by other antioxidants and can resume their function. This maintains the balance and protects healthy cells from being destroyed.

Winter swimming is a form of oxidative stress. But before you worry too much, please keep reading: antioxidants are known for having both destructive and preventive effects. The destructive aspects occur at high concentrations, while the positive preventive effects occur at low to moderate concentrations and help in the defence against infections.

So, it's good to have a strong defence, but not too strong. The question now is whether winter swimming generates a moderate or large antioxidant defence. In a study from 2013, researchers looked at a large group of winter swimmers and found significant changes in the number of red and white blood cells after a winter swimming season.

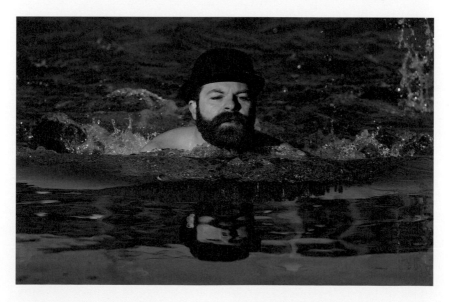

Above: A competitor takes part in the annual Fancy Dress December Dip at Parliament Hill Lido in north London, England.

According to the authors, this indicates good adaptive changes in the antioxidant system of healthy winter swimmers. The increase in antioxidants is an expression of how the winter swimmers' immune systems have improved. In addition, there was an increase in the production of antioxidants which was not accompanied by changes to other important hormones, proteins and enzymes in the body.

This is good news, as it may indicate that winter swimmers build up protection against the tissue damage caused by free radicals.

Anti-aging and winter swimming

Well, as it isn't possible to actually rejuvenate, a delaying of aging and disease might be a more accurate term. Research studies show higher levels of free radicals in the early stages of various diseases such as atherosclerosis, Alzheimer's disease and cancer. Simply by aging, our levels of free radicals increase. Yikes! I don't know about you, but I have stuff to do and no time to die. Wouldn't you like to know if we can change or delay this in some way? To some extent you can call all exercise "anti-aging" due to the anti-inflammatory effects and lower risk of disease. In the same way, winter swimming has physiological anti-inflammatory effects and could potentially lower disease risk or delay its onset, though this has not yet been proven. It is a hypothesis that should be tested by following a large group of winter swimmers over a period of many years. Such a study would provide answers to the long-term forecast for the health of winter swimmers – and may even discover that they live longer. In the light of existing research, however, it makes sense to think of winter swimming as an anti-inflammatory and immune-boosting lifestyle. I will review some of this evidence in the next section.

Winter swimming can reduce inflammation

Inflammation is the body's response to damage in tissues, muscles, tendons and ligaments, and in the bloodstream it causes atherosclerosis and increases the risk and severity of associated lifestyle diseases

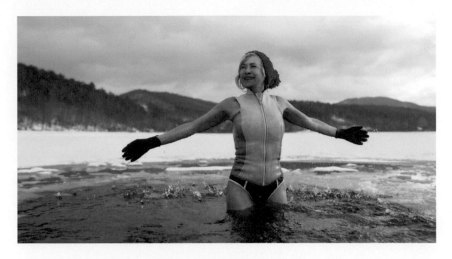

Above: A front-zipping swimsuit provides extra protection.

such as type 2 diabetes. Inflammation is a reaction triggered by the immune system, and it is scientifically proven that the inflammatory process is reduced by lifestyle changes such as eating more healthily and exercising to lower the circulating lipid – meaning cholesterol in the blood. This reduces the risk of disease and blood clots.

Could winter swimming, like exercise, lower inflammation and the risk of disease? There may well be evidence to suggest this.

We know that the immune response is improved in experienced winter swimmers, and inflammatory processes are not as pronounced, either. Studies show that swimming in cold water, like endurance exercise, has a positive effect on cardiovascular risk factors: many hormones react to cold stress, such as catecholamines (stress hormones), insulin, thyroid-stimulating hormone (TSH), adrenocorticotropic hormone (ACTH) and cortisol. Triglycerides, a type of fat/lipid found in the blood and the main components of body fat, appear to be reduced over the season in winter swimmers. Having high levels of triglycerides floating in the blood increases the risk of blood clots in the veins – so, as with bad cholesterol, it's good to keep the levels down.

As an example, a study from 2017 measured circulating lipids in the blood of thirty-four middle-aged cold-water swimmers (forty-eight to sixty-eight years old) before starting winter swimming (October), in the middle of the season (January) and after April. Triglycerides were measured in October, January and April, and the results showed lower lipid levels between January and April. A randomized controlled trial from 2014 showed improved insulin sensitivity in middle-aged men and women after seven months of winter swimming. Moreover, they found that leptin levels dropped with increased habituation to cold water. More balanced leptin and insulin levels improve the metabolism. And there are multiple studies – and therefore growing evidence – showing that experienced cold-water swimmers have lower resting blood pressure, even after just one winter swimming season. Lower blood pressure also indicates a lower degree of atherosclerosis. This can be explained by reduced inflammation in the veins and therefore less resistance for blood flow – just as water runs more smoothly in clean pipes. This, together with an improved immune system and lower lipid levels, reduces inflammation and eventually atherosclerosis.

There is an interaction between the endocrine system and inflammation. A 2000 study of long-distance cold-water swimmers showed that catecholamines (noradrenalin, adrenalin, dopamine) are lowered with cold-water habituation. I already mentioned that there are higher levels on immersion in non-acclimatized people, so let me explain:

New winter swimmers demonstrate a higher cold-shock response with a high increase in catecholamines. With habituation, the cold-shock response is lowered, also shown in the levels of catecholamines, blood pressure and heart rate. These changes are caused by the repeated activation of the central nervous system with cold water and the habituation that follows. Why? It seems plausible that lower circulating catecholamine, lipid levels, heart rate and blood pressure are results of a lower degree of inflammation in the body – an adaptation that occurs with repeated cold immersion. We need more research into the long-term effects on the immune system in experienced winter swimmers, which is why I wanted to explore this in healthy young winter swimmers. I measured their immune response in a diurnal rhythm study for twenty-four hours, compared to an equivalent non-winter-swimming control group. By measuring the circulation levels over this period we collected basic information on the blood profiles of experienced winter swimmers. With this study I believe we will have a clearer picture of the anti-inflammatory effects of cold water on the body. As this, like exercise, looks very promising, I'm sure more research exploring the health benefits will follow.

Apart from enhancing mood and energy, winter swimming can be regarded as a form of endurance exercise, or "circulation exercise", which lowers inflammation and potentially also reduces the occurrence of associated lifestyle diseases. It's a very positive add-on to any exercise regime.

Arthritis and joint pain

The acute effects of cold water are very evident – also regarding pain relief. If you talk to winter swimmers, it is not uncommon to hear them say that cold water or ice therapy has a pain-relieving effect and helps with their stiff, sore joints and arthritis pain. Surveys on motivations for winter swimming and saunas have found that winter swimmers suffering from arthritis, fibromyalgia or asthma had less pain after swimming, and experienced a general improvement in their sense of well-being. With elite athletes it has been shown that ice packs and ice baths speed their recovery from painful injuries or after exercise, as it draws lactic acid out of the muscles more quickly, making them less sore and able to heal better.

Pain significantly reduces quality of life, so if winter swimming can both reduce pain and increase well-being naturally, it is understandable that many people with joint and arthritis pain head for cold water. The physiological explanation is very likely the anti-inflammatory effects of cold-water habituation. The acute pain

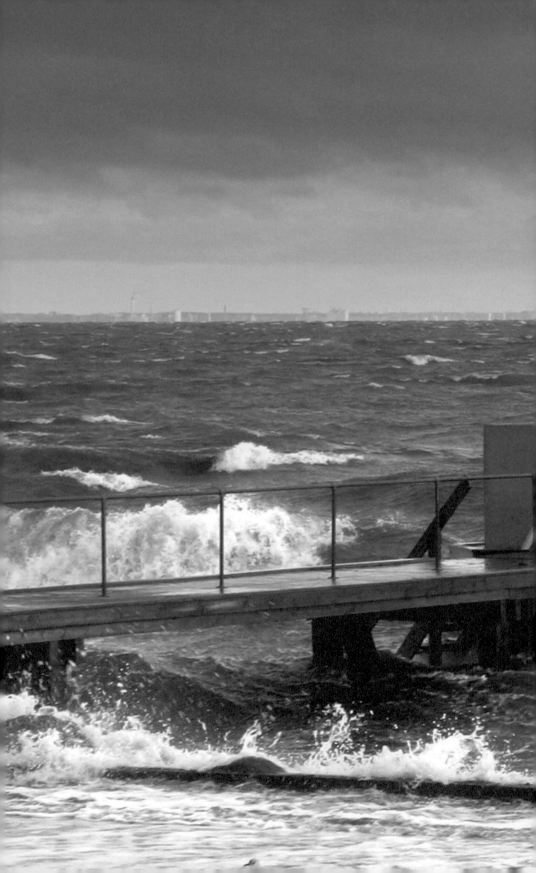

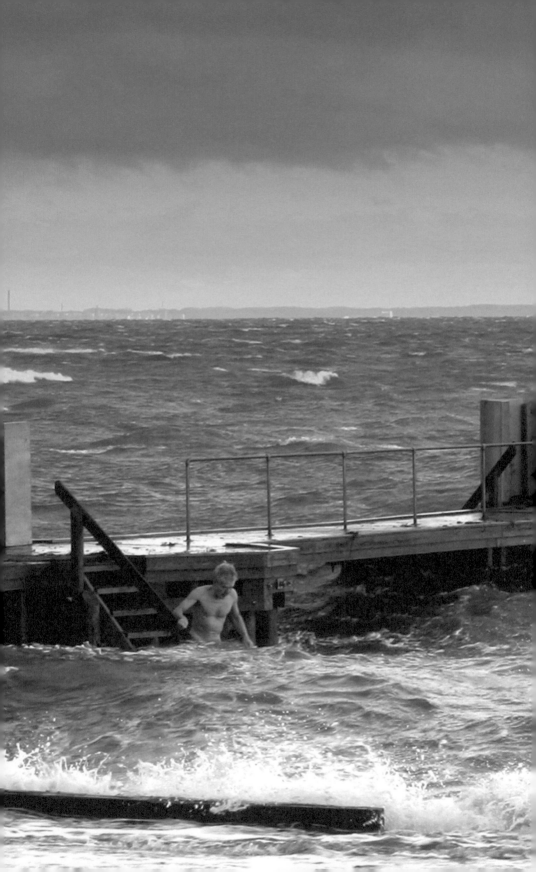

relief on entering the water is caused by nerve signalling and the release of hormones as part of the cold-shock response.

Atherosclerosis

Atherosclerosis is caused by a build-up of plaque consisting of fat, cholesterol, calcium and other substances found in the blood. Over time, the plaque hardens and narrows your arteries, which limits the flow of oxygen-rich blood to your inner organs as well as peripheral parts of your body. The deposit of fat and other substances causes an inflammatory condition, and the build-up on the inside of the artery can eventually lead to blood clots. I have seen an atherosclerotic artery in real life. It may be a little difficult to imagine what it looks like, but let me tell you – it's disgusting. Doctors and nurses among you will know what I am talking about when I tell this story.

My experience dates back many years, when I was a nursing student in the Vascular Department at Rigshospitalet and I co-assisted (or observed) during an operation. An eager and inspiring surgeon took the time after the surgery to show me an atherosclerotic blood vessel he had removed from the patient. He cut it lengthwise and – with his thumb nail! – scraaaaaped from one end of the blood vessel a thick, light-yellow and pinkish inflamed layer of fat that collected slowly but surely along his thumb. "This is a fantastic example of atherosclerosis!" he said. My eyes must have been as big as plates, and my face white. I had no doubt he was right!

The inside of the artery wall is otherwise smooth and elastic so that it can expand and adapt to large variations in blood pressure and allow blood to pass freely through the blood vessels. It is most often people with high blood cholesterol, high blood pressure, obesity, diabetes or smokers who develop severe atherosclerosis. But how does it form? First, cholesterol digs into the artery wall. The body tries to repair the damage and forms scar tissue. The vessel wall becomes thicker and

---

Pages 192–193: A "Viking" bather on the Danish coast.

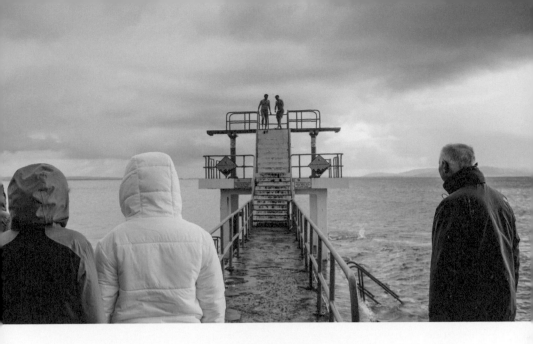

Above: The iconic Blackrock Diving Tower, Salthill, Galway, Ireland.

stiffer, and the vessel diameter – the lumen – narrower. As a result, the heart has to pump harder to force the blood through the constricted passage, and the blood pressure increases. This also explains why high blood pressure is an indicator of the health of our circulation and our atherosclerosis status. If there aren't any lifestyle changes at this stage, there is risk of a blood clot. This can most often be felt as pain, cramps and shortness of breath.

Prevention of atherosclerosis

Atherosclerosis typically occurs alongside lifestyle diseases such as diabetes and obesity. Many studies show that atherosclerosis can exacerbate complications of diabetes such as kidney failure, impaired vision and a weakened nervous system. There are also increasingly more studies showing that atherosclerosis is present in people with pre-diabetes, but it can be prevented. Not surprisingly it's about lifestyle: exercise and a low-fat diet can keep blood vessels healthy. Cut down on fatty food and get moving – walk, run, exercise – everything counts! But what about swimming in cold water? Is it healthy to expose your blood vessels to an ice-cold dip?

Winter swimming and atherosclerosis

Atherosclerosis has been measured in 115 female Japanese pearl divers who dive in cold seawater and the results compared to those of an inactive control group and a physically active control group in the same age group and from the same urban area. The question was whether diving in cold water had given the blood vessels of the pearl divers the same flexible structure and function that is found in cold-water mammals. Atherosclerosis was found to be less present in the pearl divers than in the other two groups.

As atherosclerosis is the build-up of cholesterol in the blood vessels, how can cold water reduce fat in the circulation? The cold-shock response increases energy burning to keep the body warm. This is mainly the skeletal muscles and the brown fat. The brown fat is activated by cold water and uses fuel (sugar and fat from the bloodstream) to stay activated and produce heat, thereby reducing unhealthy fat and sugar in the bloodstream. This may be one aspect in the reduction of inflammation and potentially of atherosclerosis through cold exposure.

In addition to increased fat burning, a boosted immune system is sure to decrease any inflammation. In simply mechanical terms, the passage of blood flowing in and out of the peripheral blood vessels also contributes to moving leucocytes and monocytes past areas with atherosclerosis, due to increased vascularization. The immune defence will consume the inflammation in the blood vessels, and potentially reduce atherosclerosis. This applies especially if you switch between being in cold water and a hot sauna. The cold contracts the peripheral blood vessels, and the heat of the sauna causes vasodilation.

The vascular function of winter swimmers has been trained, and accordingly they warm up more quickly than those just starting out. If you're a beginner, don't despair of ever warming up, even if you can't feel it in the beginning. If you haven't yet achieved the famous "winter swim glow" that makes seasoned swimmers' skin look so fresh, it will no doubt come if you keep it up and "exercise" your blood vessels.

Winter swimming versus exercise

The evidence for winter swimming as a "circulation exercise" is very promising, but clear evidence of the long-term effects is not yet available. Can we lose weight and burn white fat as we might with other cardiovascular exercise? The future will tell. So for now you shouldn't replace your workouts with winter swimming, but use it instead as a supplement. Winter swimming is probably too brief in duration to replace a thirty-minute cardio exercise. On the other hand, there's good evidence to suggest that even activities that don't increase your heart rate can have a beneficial effect on health, for example short and long walks. Just getting up from the chair, stretching, or in general doing small movements in everyday life may be one reason why some people are slim and others overweight. "Better a little something than nothing" has a name in this context: NEAT.

NEAT (non-exercise-activity thermogenesis) is a term for the energy you burn through the kinds of spontaneous movements you make throughout the day. You can, for example, increase your NEAT by walking to the coffee machine, walking to the bus, getting up, taking the stairs instead of the elevator and so on.

Winter swimming obviously activates your sympathetic nervous system more than NEAT and burns more energy faster. From the moment you're shivering on the jetty or poolside, your inner furnace – the brown fat and the muscles – burns energy to generate warmth to ensure survival from what your body interprets as the "dangerous experiment" of freezing in cold water. Adding winter swimming to your exercise regime might just enhance your health even more.

COLD FACTS:
WHAT DOES COLD WATER DO?

- Temporarily impairs cognitive function → meditative state.

- Increases habituation to cold → "hardening".

- Probably increases dopamine, an important hormone and neurotransmitter for well-being → happiness/good mood.

- Acutely increases endorphins, an important hormone and neurotransmitter for pain relief and mood → happiness/good mood and reduced pain.

- Acutely activates the sympathetic nervous system, which increases noradrenalin, an important hormone for activating your cold response and your healthy brown fat → energy boost! Heat! Fat burning!

Below: Sea swimming during the Winter Festival at Nauthólsvik, Reykjavik, Iceland.

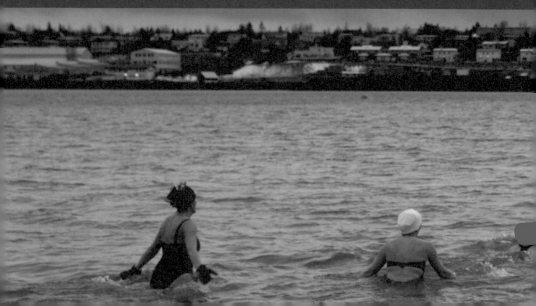

- Acutely activates the parasympathetic nervous system and stabilizes serotonin and cortisol → mental balance and potentially better sleep.

- Acutely increases noradrenalin and cortisol by activating your cold-shock response and all your muscles → readiness to fight and survive.

- Acutely increases immune response (leucocytes and monocytes) → fewer infections.

- Cold-water habituation decreases blood pressure, circulating levels of lipids, blood sugar, noradrenalin and cortisol → anti-inflammatory effect and potential reduction of atherosclerosis.

- Cold-water habituation increases insulin sensitivity → prevention of type 2 diabetes.

- Anti-inflammatory effect → reduction in swelling and joint pain.

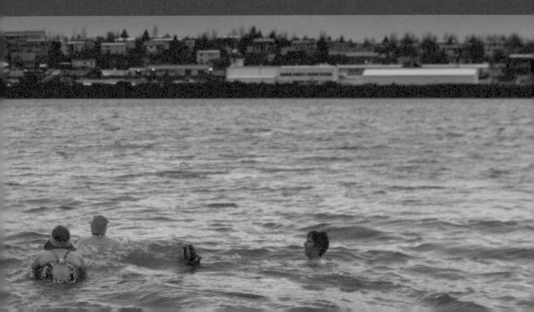

CHAPTER 11

WHAT WE CAN LEARN FROM OUR ANCESTORS

"The greater part of human misery
is due to indolence"

SAMUEL LICHTENBERG
Physicist and satirist

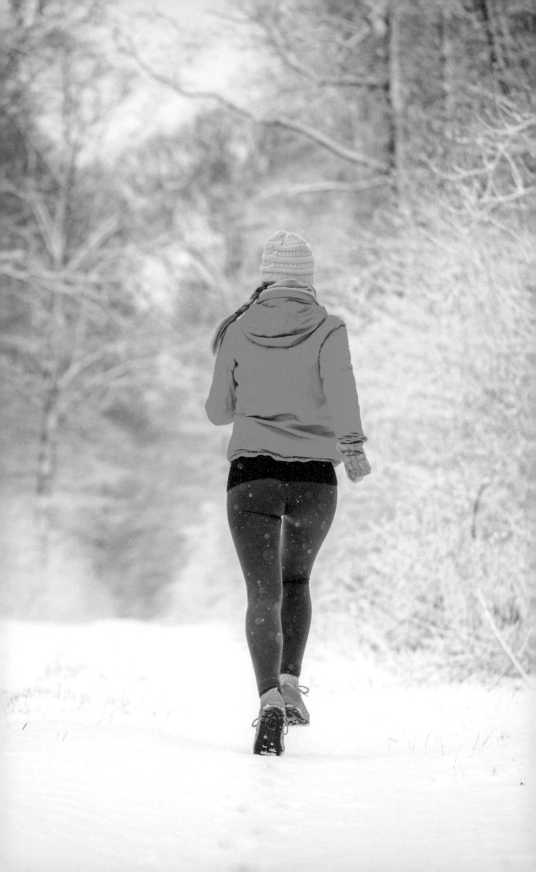

11

"IT'S WAY TOO COLD!" That's our biggest point of resistance to starting winter swimming. And it's pretty uncomfortable to be freezing cold. Having cold feet and fingers when we walk outside on a cold winter's day – the insidious cold – is a feeling we are familiar with but try to avoid. When it happens, we look forward to getting inside where it's warm, to drinking a hot cup of tea and watching a film on the sofa.

You recognize this, right? I admit that I do – I get lazy sometimes and don't like getting cold to the bone. That kind of cold doesn't give me an energy kick, or put me in a better mood. But winter swimming is a different cold – much more intense and at the same time superficial. Unlike cold wind, cold-water swimming gives warmth and energy, and puts you in a good mood. Cold water provides immediate cold over your entire body, which causes the cold-shock response and the associated activation of the sympathetic nervous system. With this kind of cold you feel a burst of inner heat, excitement and energy. So when you think, "Winter swimming is too cold for me – NO THANK YOU!" without having tried it first, you can't know whether that's true for you. Cold is cold, but cold isn't always the same kind of cold.

Our comfort has a firm grip on us all, which is why we don't seek out the challenges and physical tests that we're really built for. Just look at our ancestors, though I'm not saying we should all go out to be hunted by a bear! Luckily, there are other, safer ways: winter swimming is a controlled way to push our boundaries, which also explains why more and more people engage in it for health reasons, for an empowerment boost and as a physical challenge or social activity. Many people tell me that winter swimming has been life-changing and a starting point for a healthier way of being.

In this chapter I would like to dig a bit deeper into our psyche, to answer why it's important to break free from comfort and to mimic (to a certain extent) our ancestors' lifestyles. As you've probably guessed, winter swimming could be part of the solution.

A modern lifestyle lowers cold-induced energy burning

Most of us spend our lives finding solutions to protect our bodies from discomfort, challenges and life-threatening situations, and our bodies are weakened in the process. We live in a constant bubble of carefully controlled temperatures, from our home's central-heating system and air conditioning to the heating systems in our cars. We hardly ever take our clothes off and allow the body's largest organ, the skin, to get cold or wet, except when we shower, and even then we do it in pleasantly warm water. Winter swimming provides the ultimate cold-shock response and effectively activates our brown fat to generate heat. When we're living warmly in our houses, our body thinks there's no need for the brown fat, and it diminishes. And that's a shame, because then you have to work harder to burn off the amount of fat and sugar that the brown fat would otherwise take care of. Is it possible to change this?

By pairing your winter swimming with physical training, you're well on your way to saying goodbye to comfort and obesity. Comfort is

---

Page 202: Pair your winter swimming with a cold run.

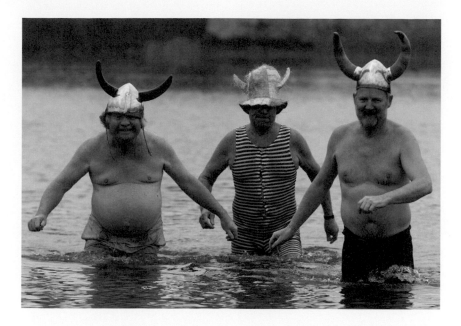

Above: Members of the Copenhagen winter swimming club *Det Kolde Gys* ("The Cold Shock") – Viking ancestry is highly likely!

unfortunately a significant killer, but there are many ways to avoid giving in to it.

One area of current research is investigating how depression is related to our sedentary lifestyle, which can lack most of the physical stressors that have been in play for much of our existence on Earth. These stressors are physical activity and short-term changes in body temperature caused by, for example, swimming in cold water or hunting for food in very hot weather – with associated frequent activation of the central nervous system.

There was probably a time when we had more natural opportunities to foster mental balance and balance in our body composition. Today we need to take active decisions to maintain our mental and physical balance. The human body prepares itself to fight, and seeks rest to build up energy for the next big fight for survival. And for all the time we're waiting, the body rests and continuously fills its energy stores. Not surprisingly the stores end up becoming too big, and we can become overweight or obese. Winter swimming is an exciting way of activating our survival instinct and the cold-shock response to affect our immune system, energy metabolism, blood circulation and mood. Cold water really knocks you out of your comfort zone. And afterwards you feel more alive than ever. You can use the energy boost to elevate yourself in spirit and channel this to do more good for yourself – maybe by going for a run or to the gym.

If you are overweight and have just begun winter swimming or exercising, you'll see things improving right away. If it takes a while before you notice results on the bathroom scales, remember that improvements in the body happen faster than can be seen by the naked eye. Every step, every short run and every swimming excursion counts.

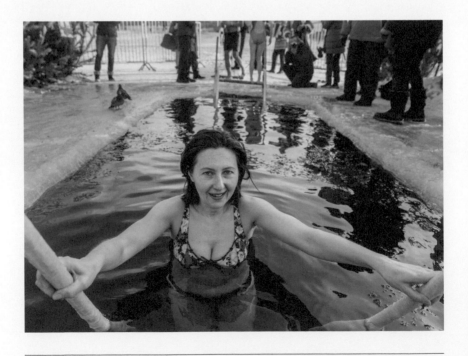

Above: A sunny day in December at the ice hole, Samara, Russia.

COLD FACTS:
MIMICKING OUR ANCESTORS

Here are some physical activities that resemble the environment of our ancestors and their daily challenges:

- Swim in cold water.

- Take a sauna.

- Run, especially in the cold. Remember, you only know it's cold if you stand still!

- Work out in the woods, preferably in the winter.

- Go hiking or take long walks in all weathers.

- Garden.

- Clean.

- Walk in the rain without a jacket.

- Sleep in a chilly room.

- Sleep in shelters outdoors, for example in the woods.

You can probably think of more challenges, ideally activities that change your body temperature. Both cold and heat challenge your health in positive ways if they are controlled and not too extreme. It requires both courage and self-discipline to voluntarily seek out situations in which we test our bodies and give them the challenges they've been created to endure.

CHAPTER 12

WINTER SWIMMING AND MENTAL HEALTH

"Happiness is the highest form of health"
DALAI LAMA
Spiritual leader

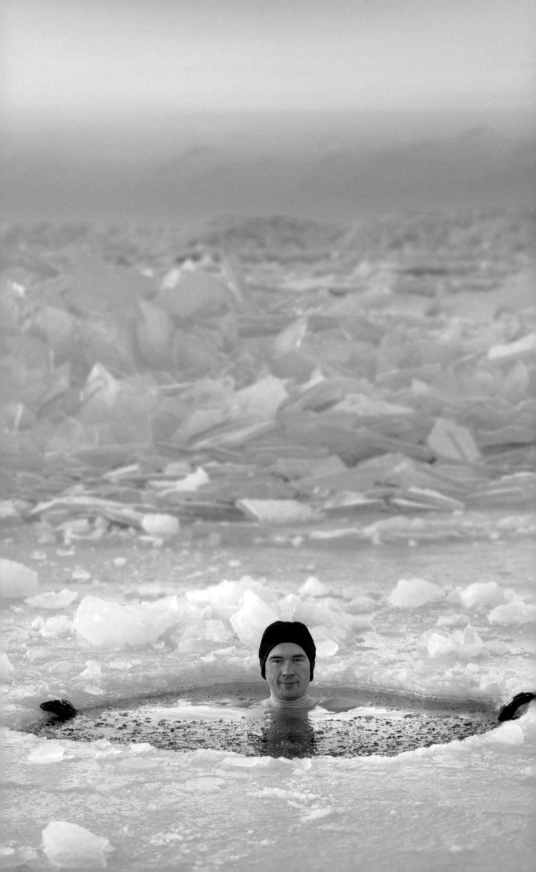

12

"Happy", "calm" and "peaceful" are often adjectives used by winter swimmers to describe the impact of winter swimming on their mental well-being. Taking into account the increase in "happiness" hormones such as noradrenalin and beta-endorphins released as part of the cold-shock response, it seems obvious to ask whether winter swimming could relieve mental disorders too.

Cold water as a treatment for depression

In a global questionnaire, winter swimmers reported an increased sense of well-being after each swim, but there are as yet no randomized controlled trials investigating the effects of winter swimming on depression or on a reduction in substance abuse. Clinical studies could provide valuable insight into how winter swimming and being out in nature can affect our mental health.

Depression is one of the leading causes of disease and disability around the world, and in 2004 was ranked by the World Health Organization as the third leading contributor to the disease burden, predicted to move to first place by 2030. And yet mental health is still a neglected area of research. Depression can affect a person's physical health, productivity, mood and behaviour and is therefore a disease that encompasses all areas of a person's life. At its worst it can be fatal. There can be no doubt that more work must be done to explore new and alternative methods to prevent and treat it.

How do we know which buttons to press to address depression? We have to go deep inside the brain where depression is born and lives ... and it begins with how the brain communicates: an imbalance in the noradrenalin signal in the brain can lead to depression. Noradrenalin works in two ways in the body – as a hormone in the blood and as a neurotransmitter in the brain, that is, as a communicator between the nerves. If noradrenalin isn't functioning properly, the brain's communication becomes defective. It has an important role in maintaining attention and focus, and increased noradrenalin in certain parts of the brain makes that region more "switched on".

So what happens in the brain when we're cold? Studies in rodents exposed to cold showed increased noradrenalin of up to four times normal levels. Repeated exposure to cold (as with winter swimmers) also provides a greater release of noradrenalin to communicate between the nerves in the locus coeruleus – the nucleus in the brain stem – which controls our reactions to stress and panic. This same significant release of noradrenalin is also found in the hippocampus (so called because its curved shape resembles a seahorse), which is responsible for human orientation and memory.

The locus coeruleus and hippocampus are both very important areas of the brain for mental health. Noradrenalin functions here alongside serotonin, and both are key signal substances – that is, "good soldiers" – that help regulate our mood. It is these exact areas of the brain and these transmitters that are targeted by many of the drugs used in the treatment of depression. It is astonishing that these specific elements in our medication can make it through such a difficult environment, namely the blood-brain barrier. This barrier is otherwise mostly closed, acting as a defensive wall to prevent the entry of pathogens and other

Page 210: Experience the glow of physical – and mental – health.

foreign elements from elsewhere in the body – we can't simply let bacteria and viruses sneak into our brains! When noradrenalin and serotonin occur naturally, i.e. not in the form of medication, they are already present in the brain and working locally to increase blood flow.

It is exciting that the cold increases noradrenalin. Consider the impact of a natural element such as cold seawater being able to improve one's mood and quality of life, by increasing neural signalling and blood flow in the brain.

But how does the brain know that it's cold? From the nerves in the skin, one of the body's first lines of defence. Upon encountering cold, our receptors will activate and send a signal to the temperature-regulating centre in the brain. Cold receptors in the skin are three to ten times more numerous than the receptors for heat. That's why we're more sensitive to cold and the body reacts quickly and intensely. So when you jump into the sea on a winter's day, it's an assault on the largest defensive walls in the body and all the cold receptors are kick-started simultaneously. It's quite overwhelming and shocking for the brain, and as a result a large and sudden onslaught of noradrenalin and serotonin is released in the body and brain at the same time. But the effect of the shock could have a positive and soothing effect on depression. In scientific literature the effect of cold water (the cold-shock response) has been likened to that of a mild electroshock treatment. Electroshock therapy is used against severe depression in some psychiatric departments.

Winter swimmers' moods

One day the research team and I were standing at the entrance to the winter swimming club in Copenhagen, talking to some swimmers who were interested in our research. A middle-aged man came over to our little group, listened for a few seconds and said, "It doesn't matter how, for me it's just healthy, I can feel it! It's working here and here!" He pointed to his heart and his head.

Winter swimming was healthy both physically and mentally, he was convinced of it. The other winter swimmers and I nodded appreciatively. For him the health benefits were a reality.

A global questionnaire also supports the subjective aspects of winter swimming. Researchers studying a group before and after four months of winter swimming found that responders felt healthier and more active and energetic than before they started. They also found that the participants had an increased sense of well-being, better memory and mood, and generally more enjoyment from life. These indicators have a great effect on one's being and one's life choices. Patients with depression often express a lack of inner calm and joy in life, diminished energy and demonstrate poorer memory. Winter swimming seems to influence exactly those areas, enhancing mood and delivering a "post-swim high", which could cause changes in behaviour and encourage us to make healthier decisions in life.

Winter swimming against depression

As mentioned, there are as yet no conclusive clinical studies investigating the effects of winter swimming on depression, but a case study from 2018 published by a research group from England describes a 24-year-old woman who had suffered from anxiety and severe depression since the age of seventeen, with symptoms such as rage, anxiety, dark moods, despair and self-harm. The usual medication for anxiety and depression did not help to ameliorate or eliminate her symptoms. Eight months after the birth of her daughter, she was anxious to be free of both her symptoms and medication.

The research team put together a programme that included swimming in a lake once or twice a week from September to April. The process of "hardening" (getting used to the cold water) and the fear of swimming outdoors were challenging for her. With the support of the researchers, she swam regularly, and gradually increased the time spent in the water as the temperature rose during spring. By the end of the following summer she could stay in the water for half an hour.

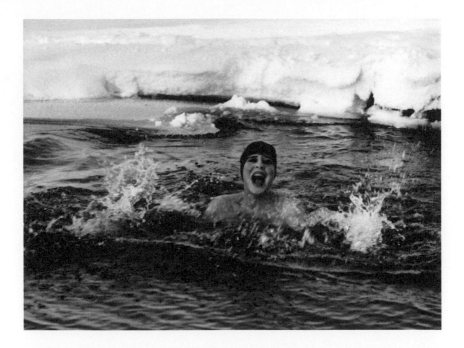

Above: In cold water, the body reacts quickly and intensely.

Every swim led to an immediate improvement of the woman's mood and a steady reduction in her symptoms of depression. From the beginning of the study her medication was gradually reduced, and four months into the trial she was no longer taking any. At a follow-up session a year later, she was still winter swimming and not on any medication.

> I really did struggle with depression and anxiety and have tried everything, CBT, talking, several different drugs and nothing worked or I feel numb and in a chemical fog. Although I didn't enjoy the cold to start with, the effect it had was like a weight being lifted off my shoulders. Open-water swimming works for me, it gets me out and about in the fresh air and has lifted my mood. I still feel down occasionally, but that is more part of what life throws my way rather than the state I was in before.
> – Tulleken et al., 2018, BMJ Case Reports

The report suggests that there are two aspects of winter swimming that work against depression: first, the physiological habituation to the cold water and the alleviation of mental stress with the cold-shock response, and second, the feeling of empowerment and achievement. It's too early for conclusions based on one case report alone, but we can wait eagerly for more evidence.

Winter swimming to combat substance abuse and addiction

On a trip to England I met two winter swimmers who had been alcoholics, and who used winter swimming as a way to reset their bodies and dampen the physical craving for a buzz or for intoxication. They explained that winter swimming had become a new habit, a way of dealing with their dependence on alcohol. They had found it a gentler replacement and managed not to drink for several years. "I drank too much," one of them said. "And I emerged from it with the help of my doctor and my wife. But I still had the urge, even though I was sober. I knew I needed more self-control, which is why I started winter swimming." What he said next was even more interesting: "It became a habit to get in the water and hang out with people at the club. And the urge to drink disappeared for a while after each swim. It was an unexpected result." The second swimmer confirmed a similar experience.

There haven't been any studies on how winter swimming might combat the urge for intoxication. But it's within the realm of possibility that the massive hormone- and neural-signalling kick triggered by cold water might quell that urge. Furthermore, the combination with the social aspect and the ability to do something else when the temptation hits are part of the explanation. When the body is alcohol-dependent, it craves a rush. The two gentlemen I met had managed to exchange that feeling for another, healthier one – they controlled their alcohol cravings with the endorphin rush of winter swimming.

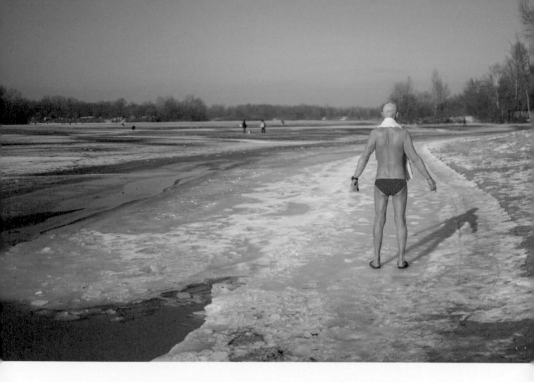

Above: Get rid of a bad habit by replacing it with a new and healthy one.

Regardless of the level of substance abuse, it requires self-control and new habits to change behaviour. If you want to get rid of a bad habit, the success rate is greatest if it is replaced by a new (healthier) habit.

So can winter swimming replace the "rewarding" and addictive effects of alcohol, drugs or gambling? I think this area of research has huge potential. It is important to note that winter swimming should not replace professional help to treat acute and severe substance abuse or depression. It is still a hypothesis, after all. The future will show to what extent, if any, cold-water therapy can be used to prevent, ameliorate or cure these conditions.

CHAPTER 13

IN THE SAUNA

"Sauna is the poor man's medicine"
FINNISH SAYING

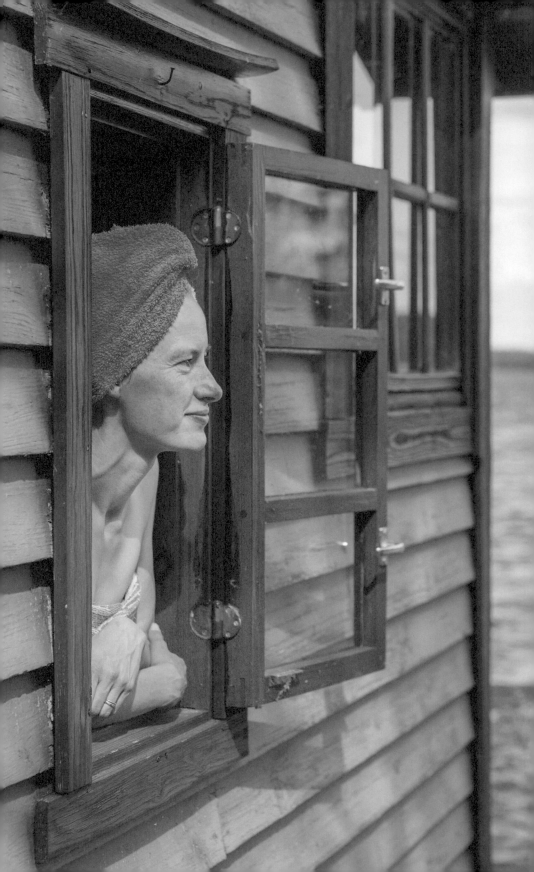

13

A sauna and a cold-water swim have become an increasingly popular wellness combination as an alternating thermal challenge. On social media the popularity becomes obvious, as people of all ages jump into cold water for cold-water dipping or ice-swimming, and warm up in a little "room of fire", a sauna hut that is stationary or on wheels. Denmark is a cold country, but we don't have a sauna tradition, whereas our Nordic neighbours have used heat therapy since antiquity. The question is whether we've been missing something; is the sauna really that healthy?

Most people have heard of Finnish saunas, where the sauna tradition has its origins and where it is a major part of the culture. According to the Finnish Ministry of Foreign Affairs, there are some two million saunas in a country with a population of 5.5 million, so even if you don't have one yourself, you can be sure one of your neighbours does! According to the Finns, a sauna is the mark of "a good home" and is used in both summer and winter as a social activity – as an icebreaker in a business context or privately with friends. "Everyone is equal in a

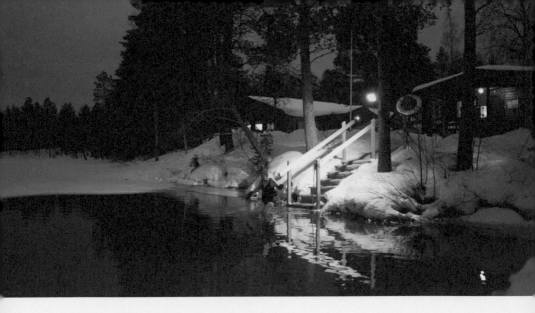

Page 220 and above: Saunas of Finland.

sauna," say the Finns. Sauna use is also widespread in Germany and Central Europe.

In many cultures throughout history there's been a practice of purifying the body with hot baths and steam, as well as with a sauna. The North American indigenous peoples made temazcal, or "sweat huts", in tents made of deer skin. These were often placed a little outside the camp, near running water, so that after the sweating session people would jump into the cold water. In Turkey and elsewhere in the Islamic world, the hammam has been used since antiquity, and was itself influence in part by Roman traditions of bathing, which involve humid and less humid steam baths, cold and hot baths, and added floral fragrances, oils and soaps. The skin was cleansed and nurtured with a paste of Mediterranean salt mixed with olive oil, essential oils and natural soap. The Romans alternated between different temperatures and levels of humidity in the saunas. And as with winter swimming and sauna, they rinsed the body in cold and hot water.

In Denmark we've been practising winter swimming since the nineteenth century, but without using the sauna. The Danes are real Vikings, after all! But times are changing and our knowledge of the benefits of controlled heat stress is increasing. The physiological healing effect after a sauna session can feel amazing, and there's rapid growth of wellness and spa culture around the world, just as with the emergence of fitness culture in the 1980s, with no signs of slowing down. Sweat lodges, Roman baths, dry sauna and saunagus are popping up more and more in Denmark, both in winter swimming clubs or on wheels. Sauna trucks are becoming quite common in Finland, and increasingly so in other countries too.

Sauna heat

The temperature in a sauna is usually just below 100°C (210°F) at the ceiling and about 40°C (105°F) at floor level, so the higher up you sit, the hotter it is. You will find the experienced "sauna surfers" on the top bench. Time spent in a sauna varies a great deal and can depend on body composition, hydration and habituation. The sauna is typically used for eight to fifteen minutes, after which you cool off in cold seawater, a shower or a tub. The process is usually repeated up to three times, but it is advised that you start with one or two sessions and increase to three as your habituation to the heat increases. Does the heat in a sauna vary during a session? In some saunas it can feel that way. In Finnish sauna and saunagus, water is poured over the hot stones, which increases humidity – it can feel like your skin is on fire!

On one of our experimental days, a participant met with us at Rigshospitalet in Copenhagen. We got into a long discussion about the effect of sauna heat, which was quite in contrast to the purpose of the day – getting cold! And we were going to measure if he had any brown fat. It was 6.30 in the morning and we were in our lab in the PET/CT Department in the basement of the hospital, setting up the day's equipment. The participant was excited and morning-fresh, and he was talking a lot. I prepared for the cooling test: blue cooling mats were laid on the bed and connected to a cooling machine, and the sterile anaesthesia table was set up. The winter swimmer then asked a good but technical question: "When you sit in the sauna and water gets poured over the heated stones, it feels like it's getting a lot hotter – is it?" At the time I didn't know, but I've since found out that two things happen: on the one hand it doesn't really get warmer, in fact it might even get a little colder as water uses up a lot of energy for evaporation. On the other hand, it feels warmer because the humidity level rises, and it becomes harder for our sweat to evaporate because the air is already saturated with water molecules. This means that the skin cannot give off sweat to cool itself down. Water molecules in the air also provide greater thermal conductivity, so the heat arrives more readily at the surface of the skin. Altogether, this will increase your skin temperature very rapidly and eventually also your core temperature.

In a dry sauna, the temperature is higher with low humidity, and so sweat is able to evaporate off the skin to cool down. In a comparative study from 2014, ten healthy males were exposed to a dry sauna versus a wet sauna for three sessions of fifteen minutes with five-minute breaks. During the breaks, the participants cooled their bodies with a cold shower. The scientists found that rectal temperature and heart rate was higher in the wet sauna, and the participants felt greater physiological stress. This makes sense, as the high humidity in a wet sauna allows for lower thermoregulation mechanisms compared to the dry sauna.

In a sauna you can tolerate something over 100°C (210°F) at moderate or low humidity. In a steam bath you would be scalded if the temperature was 100°C because the humidity is 100 per cent, so the temperature of steam baths is kept much lower, at something like 40-50°C (104-122°F). Furthermore, a thirty-minute session in a sauna heated to 80°C (176°F) causes a person's body temperature to rise by 0.9°C (1.6°F). That's a relatively high increase in temperature. It's advised to drink water before, during and after sauna sessions, and to leave the sauna straightaway if you feel uncomfortable. Be aware of signs of heatstroke: dizziness, thirst, a dry mouth, hyperventilation and/or confusion.

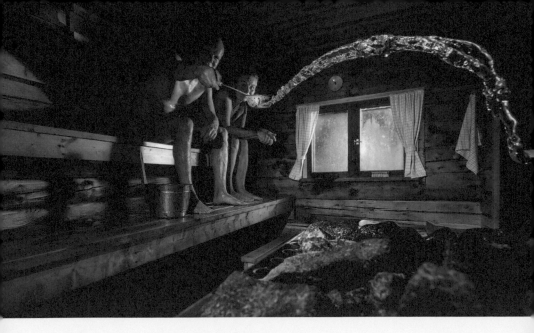

Above: More steam needed, Kuopio, Finland.

Sweating and toxins

Can you really sweat out waste products and toxins? I'm often asked this question, and now and then I hear people talk about the sauna as a place to cleanse oneself of toxins through sweating. I decided to dig into the evidence a little, to see if I could find any research on the physiology of this. In the sauna, the intense heat activates temperature receptors in the skin, which signals to the temperature-regulating centre in the brain, the hypothalamus. In the typically warm Finnish sauna, blood flow to the skin increases by 5 to 10 per cent, to avoid overheating, and the heart rate increases too, whereas blood flow to the internal organs decreases as body temperature increases.

Sweating increases the loss of water, urea, sodium, potassium, chloride, lactate and possibly other substances. A study from 2012 into the physiology of sweat-gland function suggests that the concentrations of metals and toxins present in sweat are relatively low. The amount of waste products and toxicants from sweating also seems to be minor compared with other excretion via the kidneys and gastrointestinal tract. It would probably be more cleansing to drink lots of water than to sit potentially too long in a sauna, with the

HOT FACTS:
WHEN YOU TAKE A SAUNA

- Never drink alcohol before or during a sauna. Alcohol can cause dizziness and dehydration, and unbalances the temperature-regulating centre. There is a danger of heatstroke.

- Don't wear jewellery.

- Don't use creams or lotions as they prevent the skin from breathing.

- Take a clean cotton towel to sit on, and protect your hair with a towel regardless of its length. The intense heat dries out the hair.

- Never throw water onto the sauna stones when people are sitting near them.

- Cool down after the sauna with a dip in cold water or a cold shower.

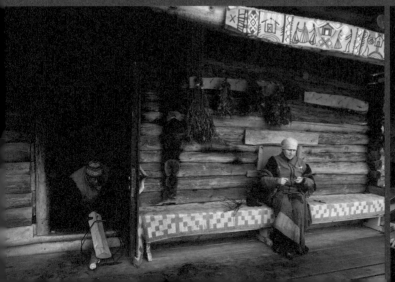
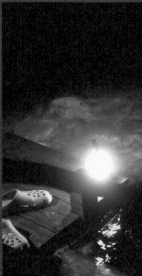

- Switch between the sauna and cold water to get the most out of a sauna experience.

- Drink plenty of cold water before, during and after the sauna to prevent dehydration.

- Do not stay in the sauna longer than fifteen to twenty minutes at a time.

- Leave the sauna immediately if you feel dizzy, nauseous or uncomfortable.

- Do not leave children or disabled people unattended in the sauna. Sauna is strictly forbidden for babies and is not recommended for younger children or pregnant women due to the risk of heatstroke.

- Avoid strenuous physical activity for at least ten minutes after a sauna.

Below: Preparations for using a smoke sauna near Haanja, Estonia. Smoke saunas are usually built without a chimney and have a stove that rests on boulders where firewood is burned until the room heats up. When the right temperature is reached and the smoke has gone, it is traditional to whisk each other with birch twigs.

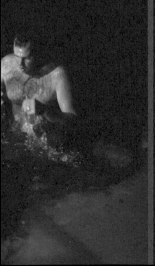
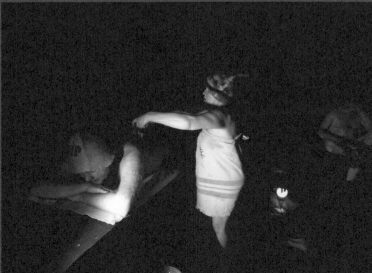

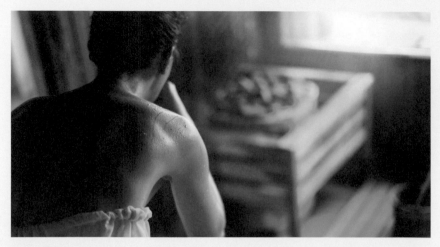

Above: Keep hydrated before, possibly during, and certainly after a sauna.

risk of dehydration and heat stroke! Further research is needed to determine whether taking a sauna is a useful strategy for excreting toxins – and more specifically how much time is needed in the heat. I cannot be sure, but I suspect it would take too long, which wouldn't compensate for the detrimental effects on the cardiovascular system and the danger of heatstroke. One good piece of advice is to keep hydrated before, possibly during, and certainly after a sauna. If you stay hydrated, the kidneys and gastrointestinal tract will take care of waste products and toxins – it's cleansing in itself.

Are saunas healthy?

"Do you know?" a middle-aged lady asks me in the lounge of the club, where I was waiting for winter swimmers from my study. She probably recognizes me from the poster about the research project on the noticeboard behind me.

"The short answer is that it's probably healthy in more or less the same way as cold is, if it's not extreme. The health benefit comes from adaptation to cold stress and heat stress," I answer. The processes behind these two work quite differently, however.

Winter swimmers are always keen to know whether cold-water swimming and sauna are healthy activities in combination, and whether they're missing out on some of the benefits in the "winter-swimming health package" if sauna is left out. Or whether the sauna is simply superfluous from a health perspective, or even whether the heat cancels out the benefits of the cold water. In the wake of the popularity of cold-water and winter swimming, these are important questions. For many, winter swimming is simply jumping into cold water, which we've been doing in Denmark since time immemorial. For others, it's the complete experience – a balance between temperatures – which ultimately constitutes the challenge and the joy of "thermal wellness".

"For me it's the interaction between contrasting temperatures," the lady in the lounge continued. "The cold and the heat belong together, just like yin and yang. I think it's good for blood circulation and for my mood. And it can be just as difficult to stand the heat of the sauna for ten to fifteen minutes as it is being in the water for a minute," she said. "These days I'm also not freezing cold all the time," she concluded. Her adaptation to the cold had increased.

Hot or cold – what feels best?

In one of my research projects, we measured the influence of cold and heat on brown-fat activity in winter swimmers and a control group. On day one, the participants were cooled for three hours using water-perfused blankets with an adjustable temperature around 12–14°C (53–57°F). The blankets were made of silicone, through which water flowed to and from a cooling/heating machine, and the aim was to balance the cooling of the participants to activate the brown fat, but also to avoid muscle shivering. On the second day, they were kept warm for three hours with water at about 32°C (90°F).

I expected that the day of cooling would be far more challenging for the participants than the warm temperature, but it turned out to be the other way around. Subjects generally found it easier to endure cold than a moderate heat over a long period.

Heat stress and habituation

It is important for the body to maintain its temperature and to avoid overheating, to keep the internal organs functioning optimally. Studies on exercising in warm temperatures show that exposure to heat can cause mild hyperthermia, i.e. an increase in the body's core temperature. A higher core temperature induces a thermoregulatory response, in which neuroendocrine, cardiovascular and protective mechanisms of proteins work together to restore homeostasis (balance). As with cold acclimatization, the body is preparing and "hardening" for future heat stressors. As well as being a "wellness" activity, sauna is also used for heat acclimatization for endurance runners, to enhance performance.

When you take a sauna, the physiological response to heat is the opposite to the response of the cold water: temperature receptors in the skin signal to the temperature-regulating centre in the hypothalamus that there is a danger of overheating. To avoid this, the veins dilate and direct the blood to the skin, where heat is released by dilation of the small capillary veins. This becomes obvious when the skin turns red and becomes warm, and the sweat glands activate. Studies in human physiology investigated the heat-stress response and the intriguing impact on hormonal changes and health. Heat stress activates the sympathetic nervous system with the same hormonal output as in the cold-shock response. But, in contrast to cold stress, the physical effects of heat are a significant increase in blood pressure and heart rate as the blood moves away from the core, in turn increasing the respiratory rate and vascularization of the skin. A literature review assessed blood flow to the skin at different temperatures in people with both high and low BMI. It seems that blood flow, as a response to acute heat stress, increases up to seven to eight litres (fifteen to seventeen pints) per minute, whereas normal blood flow to the skin is much less, though how much is still uncertain. But as mentioned above, it seems that sauna use increases blood flow to the skin in general.

Perhaps the strongest and most enduring effect of the heat-stress response is an improved perspiration capacity and lower core body temperature, which increases the body's tolerance for heat. More specifically, studies have shown that the baseline core temperature (i.e. not in the sauna) is lowered by 0.3–0.4°C (0.5–0.7°F) as a result of heat habituation. By lowering the core temperature, the body prepares for the next heat exposure and protects inner organs from overheating.

We are advised to be very careful not to stay too long in the sauna. Although acclimatization and habituation can increase the time we spend in the heat, there is a maximum threshold before our proteins begin to sustain damage. Proteins are the building blocks of our bodies, and if the body can't release heat, we begin to hyperventilate. Oxygen is absorbed by red blood cells in the lungs, and if we get too warm, we bring more oxygen into our lungs than we need, while also disposing of more carbon dioxide than normal. Increased oxygen isn't damaging, but when carbon dioxide is breathed out it leads to significant changes in our blood's acidity levels (pH), which can lead to hyperventilation. If you hyperventilate, feel tingling in your fingers, ears or eyes, it's time to get out, cool off and drink water. If you don't get out of the sauna before you feel dizzy and uncomfortable, you could lose consciousness. So don't push yourself too much – habituation is a built-up achievement.

Sauna and cardiovascular risks

There is still not a great deal of research into the effect of blood flow to the myocardium (heart musculature) during heat stress, but it is thought to increase in a similar way to that of blood flow to other muscles. If so, it's good news for people with coronary artery disease, also known as atherosclerosis. But even if we have to wait for research that delves deeply into the effects of heat stress on the heart, we can look at the long-term effects of the Finnish sauna on heart conditions.

The Finnish Kuopio Ischemic Heart Disease Risk Factor Study consisted of a population-based sample of 2,315 men from Eastern

Finland (age range forty-two to sixty years), known as the "Finnish Sauna Cohort". Baseline examinations were performed between March 1984 and December 1989, with a follow-up study in 2015 on the association of frequency/duration of sauna use with the risk of sudden cardiac death and mortality from all causes. Health examinations were performed at the onset and researchers recorded how many times a week participants went to the sauna, and for how many minutes. It was noted which of the participants subsequently had cardiovascular disease or died of heart failure.

The results showed that taking a sauna of five to eighteen minutes, four to seven times a week, was associated with a 40 per cent lower risk of death from all causes, compared to a sauna once a week or not at all. There was also a 23 per cent lower risk of coronary heart disease with sauna use two to three times per week and a 48 per cent lower risk with sauna use four to seven times a week, compared to sauna once a week or not at all. Those who used the sauna four to seven times a week had a significant reduction – 50 per cent – in their risk of death from cardiovascular disease, and those using the sauna two to three times a week had a 27 per cent lower risk, regardless of conventional risk factors.

However, researchers also found that sauna use exceeding nineteen minutes per session was associated with an increased risk of severe cardiovascular disease, but not a general increase in mortality. It seems that if the sauna isn't overused, there are associated significant and positive long-term effects on cardiovascular health. The study may also indicate that there is an upper limit of nineteen minutes, at which point the effects of the sauna become too strenuous for the cardiovascular system. Everything in moderation, the saying goes, and that's absolutely true in terms of stressors on the body.

A few years later, in 2018, the same cohort of Finnish sauna users were examined to explore an association between sauna sessions three to seven times a week with exercise twice a week and a potential link to a lower risk of death from heart failure. In this follow-up study, researchers found a link between the combined exercise and sauna regimen and a significantly lower risk of heart failure (69 per cent). Furthermore, there seemed to be a significantly lower risk of heart failure compared with groups who used the sauna or exercised less than twice a week.

In 2019, another study on the Finnish Sauna Cohort looked at sauna use and the risk of developing deep vein thrombosis (DVT, blood clots in the legs). It found an association between sauna use two to three times a week and a lower risk of DVT. The risk reduction was nearly 50 per cent compared to people taking a sauna once a week or not at all. Notably, those who used the sauna four times or more had the same risk as those who used the sauna once or not at all, which means that taking a sauna two to three times a week may reduce the risk of DVT by 50 per cent.

Yet another study of men in the same group showed a correlation with a 61 per cent reduced risk of having a new blood clot in the brain in those who had already suffered one with sauna use four to seven times a week, compared to once or not at all. This may indicate that the alternating blood flow to the brain and contraction and dilation of blood vessels in the body acts against atherosclerosis.

Exercise for the heart

Sauna causes sympathetic activation and can be seen as exercise for the heart, or cardiovascular exercise, in other words. During a sauna session, the pulse rate can reach 100 beats per minute in moderate heat and up to 150 beats per minute in very hot temperatures. Such a high heart rate corresponds to physical activity at moderate to high intensity. A 2018 study showed that even a single short session in a sauna can reset irregular heart rates, measured right after the sauna, in patients with untreated high blood pressure. Another study from Finland tested blood pressure in a hundred men and women. They found that patients with slightly raised blood pressure had lowered blood pressure measured within twenty-four hours after a single sauna session of thirty minutes. The study also showed that sauna use led to an improvement in arterial stiffness. Arterial stiffness is an indication of atherosclerosis. As increased cholesterol is associated with a higher risk of atherosclerosis, it would be interesting to investigate if lipids in the blood are altered as well.

Cholesterol and the sauna

If spending time in the sauna activates the sympathetic nervous system, increases heart rate and lowers blood pressure upon habituation, it is likely that sauna use could affect circulating cholesterol levels. A Polish study from 2014 assessed the effect of sauna use on the lipid profile and found it corresponded to the benefits achieved through moderate-intensity exercise. I find it fascinating that a passive therapy such as sauna heat can lower cholesterol levels, baseline heart rate and blood pressure upon habituation – without even having to move a muscle to increase energy expenditure! I assume that taking saunas and exercising could have a synergistic effect on health outcomes as well. This effect is perhaps what the Finnish Cohort study observed in the twenty-five-year follow up on sauna users who exercised twice a week and had an associated lower risk of heart failure and mortality. Conclusively, these studies suggest that a health regime of taking a sauna alongside exercising could indeed increase your health, and potentially your healthy life years.

The sauna and the immune system

Can sauna use boost the immune system and potentially reduce our susceptibility to colds and infection? Like winter swimming, taking a sauna raises oxidative stress by activating the sympathetic nervous system, which can lead to improved antioxidative capacity. A study from 1988 evaluated the early evidence and found that sauna use had a direct effect on the respiratory tract and lung tissue, including an improvement in breathing and lung function in patients with asthma and chronic bronchitis. A further study suggests that sauna use

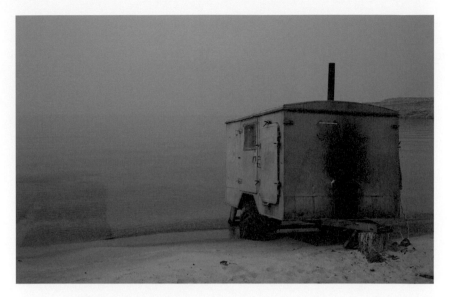

Above: A traditional sauna (*banya*) on the edge of Lake Baikal, Siberia, Russia.

improved lung function in twelve male participants with obstructive pulmonary disease, and another observed that sauna use reduced the occurrence of colds by 50 per cent.

The findings that sauna use improves symptoms of lung disease and increases lung capacity might also explain recent findings in the Finnish Sauna Cohort. In 2017 the researchers published a study showing that sauna use is associated with a reduced risk of pneumonia. They calculated the number of times participants had been hospitalized with pneumonia during the twenty-five years of the study and found that taking a sauna once a week was associated with a 31 per cent lower risk of contracting the disease, and a sauna four to seven times a week showed a 44 per cent lower risk compared to once a week or not at all. In another study from the same cohort it was found that moderate (two to three sessions a week) to high (four to seven sessions) sauna use was associated with a reduced risk of respiratory diseases such as chronic obstructive pulmonary disease, pneumonia or asthma.

It seems, therefore, that sauna use is a simple solution to swiftly improve both cardiovascular and respiratory health.

The sauna and mental health

The sauna, like cold-water swimming and exercise, is a short-term whole-body stressor with acute sympathetic activation. As exercise shows antidepressant effects, it would be interesting to look into whether sauna use can improve mental health too. In 2019, an online survey conducted across twenty-nine countries explored the physical and mental health of regular sauna users. The participants responded that they used the sauna once or twice a week on average, their main reasons being to reduce stress and pain, and to enhance their social lives. People with joint or muscle pain experienced the most significant pain relief. More than 80 per cent of the participants experienced improvement in sleep and in their overall sense of well-being. About 90 per cent reported symptoms such as dizziness, dehydration and headache, but nothing severe enough to warrant hospitalization.

Sauna use is known to promote well-being and relaxation. One explanation might involve an opioid called "dynorphin" (the opposite of endorphin), which is produced in the brain and spinal cord. When you sit in a sauna, your dynorphin levels increase. Dynorphin is responsible for dysphoria, a deep feeling of restlessness or dissatisfaction which is responsible for the body's response to heat and involved in the process of cooling the body down. Dynorphin release indicates that hyperthermia represents a form of stress. When dynorphin binds to opioid receptors, this triggers pain and distress. This doesn't sound good, does it? But interestingly the brain then increases the production of mu-opioid receptors that sensitize the brain to endorphin exposure in the future. So even though at first it doesn't feel good sitting there in the sauna sweating, it makes your brain more sensitive to endorphins – one of our happiness hormones. Exposure to sauna heat is a natural painkiller, which explains why we feel better and better with sauna use, and why we observe an increase in well-being, mental balance and a feeling of happiness in the longer term.

A follow-up study on the Finnish Sauna Cohort investigated how sauna use relates to the development of mental disorders such as dementia, Alzheimer's disease and psychosis, and the results suggest a reduced risk of diseases of the nervous system. Sauna use four to seven times a week appears to reduce the risk of dementia by 66 per cent and Alzheimer's disease by 65 per cent as compared to those using the sauna only once a week or not at all. The same research group investigated a link between sauna use and the risk of psychosis in men who had not been psychotic in the past. The results suggests that sauna use four to seven times a week led to a 23 per cent lower risk of psychosis compared to sauna use only once a week or not at all. Psychosis is a condition which is triggered by other disorders such as schizophrenia, schizophrenic disorders, delusions and depression. It is possible that the alternating of heat and cold and blood supply to and from the brain could have positive mental-health effects.

This rather condensed summary suggests that the sauna is definitely worth considering, if or whenever possible, as part of your healthy lifestyle and winter-swimming regime.

Essential oils

December was cold and dark. We, the team from the winter-swimming science project, wanted to go on a work outing – something special, and well deserved, too! A place where we could relax . . . so we went to Amager to try out a Native American sweat lodge beside the water. The purification ritual performed is called inípi, and participants seek to enter a state of humility, and to undergo a kind of spiritual rebirth. The sweat lodge is central to inípi.

We were looking forward to the feeling of warmth, cold and not least the experience of saunagus and all that it entails. Most of us hadn't tried it before, so we were excited. We put on our swimwear, and the gus master waved us into a place shaped like a little igloo. It looked authentic. There was a small, low entrance with a leather blanket to cover it, and once we were inside, the "igloo" was not tall enough to stand up in. The gus master let the blanket down and we were in the dark. We sat quietly on tiny benches with twenty other

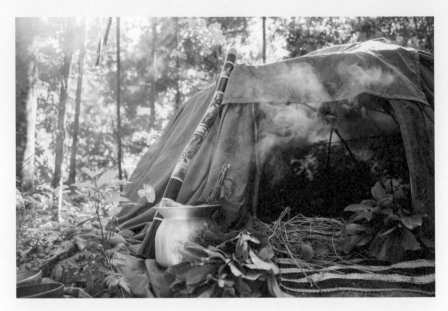

Above: A Native American sweat lodge.

heat-craving people. The gus master introduced first one, and then another essential oil, and ladled cold water onto a large stove in the middle of the small hut. It got so hot that some people had to leave. As we sat in the oil-infused steam, he told us of each oil's positive effect on our health.

"This one's peppermint – it works well for . . ." he'd explain, "and lavender's particularly good for . . ."

"Is it really healthy?" one of the girls whispered to me.

I didn't know; it was a good question!

"Now it's time to go in the water," he said, lifting the blanket away from the little entrance. The heat rolled out along with waves of steam into the icy air, while all the participants, red as crayfish, poured out with it. The air was thick with anticipation – we were heading for the water!

In a saunagus session, the gus master pours different essential oils, one by one, over hot lava rocks. One oil is said to be good for blood circulation, others for the immune system, and so on. But are there really any health benefits from inhaling the oil-infused vapour? Many people believe that essential oils can help in the treatment of diseases of the upper and lower respiratory tracts. But, as far as I know, there is no scientific documentation on the beneficial effects of essential oils on health – nor in combination with heat. In a 2018 study of 106 participants, researchers investigated the effects of peppermint, eucalyptus and rosemary oil on lung function. Participants were randomly selected to inhale one of the three types of oil, or no oil at all, for fifteen minutes. The results showed that none of the oils had a measurable effect on various lung-function measurements. Furthermore, the researchers found that the subjects' perceived expectations of better lung function and the measurable effects were not in sync.

Does this mean that essential oils don't work? Probably not, at least not for the improvement of lung function or blood circulation. It is possible, however, that essential oils work indirectly on our ability to relax. The oils are sensory stimulators which we associate with relaxation and personal care. In the same category, we have scented massage oil, shampoo, soaps and creams. The brain connects the scents with relaxation because they have always been associated with the cleansing of the skin and relaxation, with associations to ancient bathing rituals. That's how it's always been – your brain immediately recognizes the pleasant fragrances and you automatically take a deep breath and relax in the sauna. The oils give the brain something specific and sensual to focus on, and can have an indirect positive influence on well-being and stress reduction. It's a desirable placebo effect.

"Make time to go into the sauna," a winter swimmer kindly advised me. "Sometimes you have to relax mentally and 'empty your brain'."

It's a piece of advice I've taken to heart – and preferably with the help of essential oils.

Pages 240–241: Early morning mist on Lake Gåxsjön, Sweden.

HOT FACTS:
HEALTH BENEFITS OF THE SAUNA

- Lowers blood pressure and heart rate. Reduces the risk of cardiovascular disease, possibly due to less overall inflammation in the body, which reduces atherosclerosis.

- Reduces the risk of dementia.

- Reduces the risk of lung disease.

- Increases well-being and calm. Promotes a healthy mental balance due to endorphins.

- May lower the risk of death from heart failure and other causes when used more than once a week for a maximum of nineteen minutes per session.

- May lower risk of death from heart failure further if cardiovascular exercise twice a week is combined with sauna use three to seven times a week.

- May reduce the risk of blood clots by 50 per cent with sauna use three to four times a week.

HOT FACTS:
THE SAUNA CAN BE DANGEROUS

- If you don't listen to your body's signs of overheating – a tingling in the fingers, ears and skin, and/or hyperventilating.

- If you don't drink enough water before, during and after the sauna.

- If you have been drinking alcohol.

- If you suffer from cardiovascular disease, irregular heart rate, high or low blood pressure, fever, cancer, skin disorders (with or without inflammation), or are in treatment for blood clots or varicose veins.

- If you have respiratory infections.

- If you take medicines that can activate the sympathetic nervous system, as they can induce cardiac arrhythmia.

If you are uncertain your condition or medication allows you to use a sauna, consult a doctor.

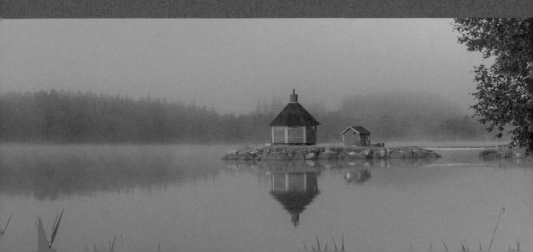

AFTERWORD

The popularity of cold-water swimming and taking saunas are good examples of the current wellness wave. This isn't simply wellness as we've known it, with yoga, massage, meditation, steam baths and so on. No, this is a kind of "nature wellness" which integrates nature as part of a physical and mental health regime. Interest has increased over the past five years, but the enthusiasm for winter swimming has surged during the Covid-19 pandemic and consequent lockdowns around the world. During these daunting times, people who may already have aspired to become a winter swimmer suddenly had the time to try. People were looking for excitement, kicks and laughs in a depressing time. A dip in open water or the sea to enhance happiness is accessible and costs nothing. And as I write these final words, lockdowns are still restricting our daily lives.

For the last six years, throughout my research into brown fat and winter swimming, people have reached out to me on social media and sent me fascinating and touching "swim stories". They tell me how winter swimming has changed their lives and saved their mood in lonely times – and especially lately during the pandemic. The love for cold water has made headlines on TV and in newspapers, and on social media the popularity is plain to see. Even our former prime minister of Denmark, Helle Thorning-Schmidt, can be seen on Instagram dipping elegantly into "slush ice" with a huge smile. She, along with many others, had her winter-swimming debut during a Covid-19 lockdown. Here's another:

I never ever thought I was going to be a winter swimmer.
I consider those who swim in freezing-cold water half crazy.
The sea temperature at the beginning of the summer had
always been (more than) abundantly cold for me. Then came
the pandemic. After ten months of Corona prison my girlfriend
and I had gone crazy enough, and one icy January day we

challenged each other to jump into the sea. And we did. And it was WILD. It was incredible how many different sensations I experienced in my body in the few seconds it took to get into the water and quickly back out onto the jetty. I felt a cold against my skin, sharper than I had ever experienced before. And then an amazing inner warmth that I had never felt before. And throughout the episode, a sense of euphoria and presence in the now. When we sat in the car afterwards, drinking a cup of coffee, and talked about our experience, we had no doubt that it should be repeated.

– Anders, first season, 29, Denmark

Many people I've spoken to say that their tolerance of rain and cold weather is much improved after becoming a winter swimmer, and even express an excitement for outdoor life. Nature, with its simple but harsh presence, does not deceive, as opposed to the internet and social media and their endless guides and "advice". Nature is sincere; it's neither for nor against us. Our winter-swimming expedition is, however, conditioned by the physical environment in which we swim, so a respect for nature is essential.

Do you look for ways to increase your energy levels, to feel more balanced or achieve greater inner strength? Thinking back on the scientific studies mentioned in this book, it becomes clear that winter swimming is a way of empowering yourself. You don't have to overdo it to make it matter or to gain the health benefits. This is actually my favourite part: winter swimming seems to be beneficial in multiple ways, on the physical, mental and social parameters – for many people, it's a holistic way to good health.

Cold and hot temperatures are stressors that increase habituation. Cold exposure increases metabolism and activates brown fat. Brown fat and skeletal muscles produce heat by burning energy, which improves insulin sensitivity. In my studies I investigated young, healthy winter swimmers (who also use the sauna) compared to a BMI, age, sex and fitness level-matched control group. I addressed the effects of winter swimming combined with sauna use on brown fat in both cold and warm temperatures, energy metabolism in cold temperatures, the immune system, diurnal rhythmicity in brown fat, and circulating leptin and cortisol levels during the day and night.

Regular winter swimming has been shown to have a positive effect on various systems including the cardiovascular system, the endocrine system, the immune system and the psyche. However, swimming in cold water still poses a significant health risk to inexperienced swimmers and people with heart disease. To take full advantage of the metabolic effects and cold habituation requires patience and an acclimatization programme that is preferably carried out under the guidance and supervision of others. And a reminder: never swim alone. Winter swimming should always be considered a sport to do with others.

Research into saunas and health show a link to reduced mortality, and a reduced risk of depression and brain disorders such as dementia, Alzheimer's disease and psychosis. In the field of science, the cold-shock response is sometimes compared to a mini electroshock therapy, which has been shown to reduce depression. A winter swimmer described it like this:

> I have a very busy life, I'm a manager with my own business,
> I have a wife who has been in an accident . . . My head is
> constantly filled with thoughts and worries. But after a swim
> in cold water, it's cleaned up. There are absolutely no buzzing
> thoughts – it gives me a CTRL+ALT+DEL . . . and my head is as if
> reborn.
>
> – Thomas, first season, 39, Sweden

Cold-water swimming and the heat of the sauna enhance our health, especially when combined with exercise. Impressively, our ancestors already knew (or felt) the benefits of cold and hot therapies, long before we could measure them in modern times. Today, these benefits have been rediscovered, and after years of research into this topic, I firmly believe it's a healthy investment. You don't have to be Elsa to embrace the cold as there is no magic cure to good health, and it doesn't have to be overly complicated, either. Trust yourself. Listen to your body while challenging yourself in the process and it will take you anywhere! One way to increase your strength is to go back to basics, to increase your physical and mental health; swim in very cold water, take a sauna, go for a run, eat carrots and drink lots of water! It's cleansing, raw and simple. And it just takes a little courage . . .

> I hadn't been in the sea for probably fifteen years, not even in the summer, as I felt it was just too cold. I was prompted to start winter swimming due to chronic pain as a result of a traffic accident in June 2018. After various attempts at rehabilitation at the Centre for Brain Injury, the neo-optometrist, the physiotherapist, neurologist etc., my progress came to a halt and I got no better, but still suffered from the now chronic consequences of the accident. I was challenged to try winter swimming – partly by a friend who wanted company, and partly by a brain specialist. I had nothing to lose and everything to win. So on 2 January 2019, I went into the sea for the first time in many years. There was snow on the jetty. It was cold. It was beautiful. And it was a little scary. But the transformation, by walking into the water, was nothing short of absolutely wildly amazing! The woolly feeling I have in my head disappeared for a while. It was like feeling alive again. I could think better, and my speech became clearer.
>
> – Alice, second season, 54, Denmark

Every winter swimmer has their own reasons for taking up the sport, and every story is unique. For me as a scientist, listening to these stories has made the science meaningful and important.

ACKNOWLEDGEMENTS

Huge thanks to Forlaget Grønningen 1 for giving me the opportunity to communicate the thrust of more than six years of research and participation in winter swimming, and for their great editorial work and efforts with the book in all its forms.

Thanks to my doctoral advisor, Bente Klarlund Pedersen, who, out of the kindness of her heart spent time on weekends reading through this book. Her contribution and that of other researchers to knowledge sharing is a huge inspiration for scientific collaboration. Also thanks to my PhD supervisor, Camilla Scheele, for her support throughout this book project.

Many thanks to those who took part in the experiments behind the book, and to the winter-swimming association Det Kolde Gys ("The Cold Shock") at Helgoland, Copenhagen. Thank you for your invaluable efforts, which are crucial for this research to progress. Thanks also to the Novo Nordisk Foundation for supporting my research into winter swimming and brown fat.

This book would never have come together without my dedicated team of colleagues: Berenice Sevilla Moreno, Laura Aagaard, Clara Borch Jensen, Ida Elkjær and Natja Launbo. Berenice is a thesis student hailing from warm Mexico. She returns there, where a PhD position awaits her, with many memories. Thank you, Berenice, for your courage and curiosity. I'd like to cite her here:

When I heard about winter swimming in Denmark, I was surprised by the description of the activity and curious as to why anyone would volunteer to take a dip in very cold water on an already VERY cold day. I could not imagine a single reason for doing something like that, because in Mexico any day that's twenty degrees is already considered a cold day. But by learning about the social, psychological and physiological effects of winter swimming, I was finally able to convince myself to try it. Everyone came along [the team] when I took the cold dip, it made me smile and laugh so much – and in good company with friends. I will definitely try it again!

Thank you, too, to translator Dr Elizabeth DeNoma, and to Katharina Bielenberg, my publisher at MacLehose Press, for helping get my material ready for all the winter swimmers in the English-speaking world. For me this is a dream come true, to be able to communicate the benefits of science and expand our knowledge on longevity.

A special thank you to my husband, Lars – the engineer – who has diligently and patiently listened, read, commented . . . and along with our two boys Felix and Elliot, been an enormous support throughout the entire process.

Susanna Søberg

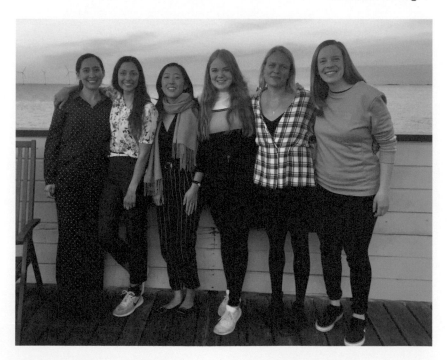

Above: The team (left to right); Berenice, me, Laura, Clara, Ida and Natja.

REFERENCES

Chapter 1

Forrester, J.M., "The Origins and Fate of James Currie's Cold Water Treatment for Fever", *Med Hist*, 2000 Jan; 44(1):57–74

Parr, S., *The Story of Swimming* (Stockport: Dewi Lewis Publishing, 2011)

Tipton, M.J., *Cold water immersion*. Chapter 6: "The Science of Beach Lifeguarding", ed. Tipton M.J. & Wooler A. (London: CRC Press, Taylor & Francis, 2016)

History of Swimming: http://www.cismeurope.org/history-swimming/

Chapter 2

Giesbrecht, G.G., "Cold stress, near drowning and accidental hypothermia: A review", *Aviat Space Environ Med*, 2000 Jul, Review

International Lifesaving Federation: https://www.ilsf.org/drowning-prevention/

Chapter 3

Hennau, Marc, "Traversée de la Meuse à la nage", Fundet, 11 August 2019

Keh, Andrew, "For Swimmers With Ice Water in Their Veins, an Event to Match", *New York Times*, 19 August 2019

Szymusiak, R., Body temperature and sleep. *Handb Clin Neurol* 2018. Review.

Tipton, M.J., et al.: "Cold water immersion: kill or cure?", *Exp Physiol*, 2017 Nov 1

Ward, Clarissa, "Ice Swimming With 'Walruses' in Russia", ABC News, 11 August 2019

Watson, Leon, "Come on in, the water's lovely! Hundreds of Russian Orthodox Christians plunge into icy pool to celebrate baptism of Jesus", *Daily Mail*, London, 11 August 2019

"Welcome to Coney Island Polar Bear Club", Coney Island Polar Bear Club, 9 September 2019

International Winter Swimming Association: https://iwsa.world/water-classification

Chapter 4

Giesbrecht, G.G., "Cold stress, near drowning and accidental hypothermia: A review", *Aviat Space Environ Med*, 2000 Jul, Review

Hartwig, A.C., Peripheral beta-endorphin and pain modulation. Anesth Prog. 1991. Review

Jones, D.M. et al: "Cold acclimation and cognitive performance: A review" *Auton Neurosci*. 2017 Dec

www.respektforvand.dk

Tipton, M.J., *Cold water immersion*. Chapter 6: "In The Science of Beach Lifeguarding", ed. Tipton M.J. & Wooler A. (London: CRC Press, Taylor & Francis, 2016)

Tipton, M.J., et al., "Cold water immersion: kill or cure?", *Exp Physiol*, 2017 Nov 1

Chapter 5

Barwood, M.J., et al., "Habituation of the cold shock response is inhibited by repeated anxiety: Implications for safety behaviour on accidental cold water immersions", *Physiol Behav*, May 2017

Bleakley, C.M., et al., "What is the biochemical and physiological rationale for using cold-water immersion in sports recovery?", A systematic review, *Br J. Sports Med*, 2010 Feb

Hartwig, A.C., "Peripheral beta-endorphin and pain modulation", *Anesth Prog*, 1991, Review

Huttunen, P., H. Rintamaki and J. Hirvonen, "Effect of regular winter swimming on the activity of the sympathoadrenal system before and after a single cold water immersion", *Int J Circumpolar Health*, 2001. 60(3): pp. 400–406

Jameson, J., Fauci, A.S., Kasper, D.L., Hauser, S.L., Longo, D.L., Loscalzo, J. eds. "About Pain receptors and Endorphins"; Rathmell, J.P., Fields, H.L., "Pain: Pathophysiology and Management"; Loscalzo, Joseph, et al., "Basic Biology of the Cardiovascular System"; Jameson, J. Larry., "Mechanisms of Hormone Action" in *Harrison's Principles of Internal Medicine*, 20th edition (New York, NY: McGraw-Hill, 2018)

Johnson, D.G., et al., "Plasma norepinephrine responses of man in cold water", *J Appl Physiol Respir Environ Exerc Physiol*, 1977. 43(2): pp. 216–220

Leppaluoto, J., et al., "Effects of long-term whole-body cold exposures on plasma concentrations of ACTH, beta-endorphin, cortisol, catecholamines and cytokines in healthy females", *Scand J Clin Lab Invest*, 2008. 68(2): pp. 145–153

Mantoni et al., "Reduced cerebral perfusion on sudden immersion in ice water: a possible cause of drowning", *Aviat Space Environ Med* 2007 Apr, 78(4): pp. 374–376

Shevchuk, N.A., "Adapted cold shower as a potential treatment for depression", *Med. Hypotheses* 2008, 70, pp. 995–1001

Sramek, P., et al., "Human physiological responses to immersion into water of different temperatures", *Eur J Appl Physiol*, 2000. 81(5): pp. 436–442

Tipton, M.J., "The concept of an 'integrated survival system' for protection against the responses associated with immersion in cold water", *J R Nav Med Serv*, 1993

Tipton, M.J., et al., "Cold water immersion: kill or cure?", *Exp Physiol*, 2017 Nov 1

Vaswani, K.K. et al., "Cold swim stress-induced changes in the levels of opioid peptides in the rat CNS and peripheral tissues", *Pharmacol Biochem Behav*, 1988

Vybiral, S., et al., "Thermoregulation in winter swimmers and physiological significance of human catecholamine thermogenesis", *Exp Physiol*, 2000, 85(3): pp. 321–326

Endorphins: *Encyclopædia Britannica*, inc. Endorphins URL: https://www.britannica.com/science/endorphin

Noradrenalin: URL: https://www.britannica.com/science/norepinephrine (Set 1. October 2019)

Chapter 6

Buijze, G.A., et al., "The Effect of Cold Showering on Health and Work: A Randomized Controlled Trial", *PLoS One*, 2016 Sep

Cannon, B., et al., "Brown Adipose Tissue: Function and Physiological Significance", *Physiol Rev*, 2004

Contreras, C., et al., "Hypothalamus and Thermogenesis: Heating the BAT, Browning the WAT", *Mol Cell Endocrinol*, 2016 Dec.

Contreras, C., et al. "Traveling From the Hypothalamus to the Adipose Tissue: The Thermogenic Pathway", *Redox Biol*, 2017

Cox, S.C., et al., "Showers: From a Violent Treatment to an Agent of Cleansing", *Hist Psychiatry*, 2019 Mar; 30(1), pp. 58–76

Eglin, C.M., et al., "Repeated Cold Showers as a Method of Habituating Humans to the Initial Responses to Cold Water Immersion", *Eur J Appl Physiol*, 2005 Mar

Flier, Jeffrey S., et al., "Pathobiology of Obesity", *Harrison's Principles of Internal Medicine*, 20th Edition, Eds. Jameson J., et al. (New York, NY: McGraw-Hill, 2018)

Forrester, J.M. "The Origins and Fate of James Currie's Cold Water Treatment for Fever", *Med Hist*, 2000 Jan; 44(1), pp. 57–74

Himms-Hagen, J., "Non-Shivering Thermogenesis", *Brain Res Bull*, 1984 Feb

Petrofsky, J.S., "Resting Blood Flow in the Skin: Does it Exist, and What is the Influence of Temperature, Aging, and Diabetes?", *J Diabetes Sci Technol*, 2012 May, Review

Shevchuk, N.A., "Adapted Cold Shower as a Potential Treatment for Depression", *Med Hypotheses*, 2008; 70(5): pp. 995–1001, Epub 2007 Nov 13

Sirgy, M.J., "Positive Balance: A Hierarchical Perspective of Positive Mental Health", *Qual Life Res*, 2019 Jul; 28

Tipton, M.J., et al., "Cold Water Immersion: Kill or Cure?", *Exp Physiol*, 2017 Nov 1

Van der Lans, A.A., et al., "Cold Acclimation Recruits Human Brown Fat and Increases Non-Shivering Thermogenesis", *J Clin Invest*, 2013

www.dgi.dk

www.risf.dk

www.iwsa.world

www.internationaliceswimming.com

Chapter 7

Arhire, L.I., et al., "Irisin: A Hope in Understanding and Managing Obesity and Metabolic Syndrome", *Front Endocrinol* (Lausanne), 2019 Aug

Cannon, B., et al., "Brown Adipose Tissue: Function and Physiological Significance", *Physiol Rev*, 2004

Contreras, C., Nogueiras, R., Diéguez, C., Medina-Gómez, G., López, M., "Hypothalamus and Thermogenesis: Heating the BAT, Browning the WAT", *Mol Cell Endocrinol*, 2016 Dec

Contreras C., et al., "Traveling from the Hypothalamus to the Adipose Tissue: The Thermogenic Pathway", *Redox Biol*, 2017

Cuevas-Ramos, D., et al., "Fibroblast Growth Factor 21 and Browning of White Adipose

Tissue", *Front Physiol*, 2019 Feb

Cypess, A.M., et al., "Activation of Human Brown Adipose Tissue by a Beta3-Adrenergic Receptor Agonist", *Cell Metab*, 2015

Cypess, A.M., et al., "Identification and Importance of Brown Adipose Tissue in Adult Humans", *N Engl J Med*, 2009

Hanssen, M.J., et al., "Short-Term Cold Acclimation Recruits Brown Adipose Tissue in Obese Humans", *Diabetes*, 2016

Hanssen, M.J., et al., "Short-Term Cold Acclimation Improves Insulin Sensitivity in Patients with Type 2 Diabetes Mellitus", *Nat Med*, 2015

Harms, M., et al., "Brown and Beige Fat: Development, Function and Therapeutic Potential", *Nat Med*, 2013

Lee, P., et al., "Temperature-Acclimated Brown Adipose Tissue Modulates Insulin Sensitivity in Humans" *Diabetes*, 2014

Scheele, C., et al., "Metabolic Regulation and the Anti-Obesity Perspectives of Human Brown Fat", *Redox Biol*, 2017 Aug

Van der Lans, A.A., et al., "Cold Acclimation Recruits Human Brown Fat and Increases Non-shivering Thermogenesis", *J Clin Invest*, 2013

Van Rooijen, B.D., et al., "Imaging Cold-Activated Brown Adipose Tissue Using Dynamic T2*-weighted Magnetic Resonance Imaging and 2-deoxy-2-[18F] Fluoro-D-Glucose Positron Emission Tomography", *Invest Radiol*, 2013. 48(10): pp. 708–14

Wu, J., Boström, P., et al., "Beige Adipocytes Are a Distinct Type of Thermogenic Fat Cell in Mouse and Human", *Cell*, 2012

https://www.who.int/health-topics/diabetes

Chapter 8

Davis R., et al., "Theories of Behaviour and Behaviour Change Across the Social and Behavioural Sciences: A Scoping Review", *Health Psychol*, Rev. 2015

Korhonen, N., "The Sauna – A Sacred Place", Universitas Helsingiensis, 4/1998, Helsinki University, Helsinki

Medlock S., et al., "Health Behaviour Theory in Health Informatics: Support for Positive Change", *Stud Health Technol Inform*, 2019 Jul

Sirgy, M.J., "Positive Balance: A Hierarchical Perspective of Positive Mental Health", *Qual Life Res*, 2019 Jul; 28

Valtakari, P., "Finnish Sauna Culture – Not Just a Cliché. The Finnish Sauna Society", https://www.sauna.fi/in-english/finnish-sauna-culture/

Webb, T.L., et al., "Using Theories of Behaviour Change to Inform Interventions for Addictive Behaviours", *Addiction*, 2010 Nov

www.vinterbader.com

Chapter 9

Brenke, R., Warnke, C.K., Conradi, E., "Heat regulation in winter swimming (ice-bathing) [German]", *Z. Physiother.*, 1985, 37, 31–36

Castellani, J.W., Young, A.J., Kain, J.E., Rouse, A., Sawka, M.N., "Thermoregulation During Cold Exposure: Effects of Prior Exercise", *J. Appl. Physiol.*, 1999, p. 87,pp. 247–252

Fainer, D.C., Martin, C.G., Ivy, A.C., "Resuscitation of dogs from fresh water drowning", *J. Appl. Physiol.*, 1951, 3, 417–426

Inoue Y., et al., "Thermoregulatory responses of young and older men to cold exposure" *Eur J Appl Physiol Occup Physiol*, 1992

Keatinge, W.R., Coleshaw, S.R.K., Millard, C.E., Axelsson, J., "Exceptional Case of Survival in Cold Water", *Br. Med. J. (Clin. Res.)* 1986, 292, pp. 171–172

Keatinge, W.R., Evans, M., "The Respiratory and Cardiovascular Response to Immersion in Cold and Warm Water", *Q. J. Exp. Physiol. Cogn. Med Sci.*, 1961, p. 46, pp. 83–94

Knechtle, B., Rosemann, T., Rüst, C.A., "Ice swimming and changes in body core temperature: A case study", *SpringerPlus* 2015, 4

Lounsbury, D.S., DuCharme, M.B., "Arm Insulation and Swimming in Cold Water", *Eur. J. Appl. Physiol.*, 2008, 104, 159–174

Mercer, J.B., "Cold – an underrated risk factor for health", *Environ Res*, 2003 May, Review

Miller, A.H. et al., "The role of inflammation in depression: from evolutionary imperative to modern treatment target", *Nat Rev Immunol*, 2016

Quan, L., Mack, C.D., Schiff, M.A., "Association of water temperature and submersion duration and drowning outcome", *Resuscitation* 2014, 85, 790–794

Rüst, C.A., Knechtle, B., Rosemann, T., "Changes in body core and body surface temperatures during prolonged swimming in water of 10°C – A case report", *Extrem. Physiol. Med.*, 2012, 1

Shattock, M.J., Tipton, M.J., "'Autonomic conflict': A different way to die during cold water immersion?", *J. Physiol.* 2012, 590, 3219–3230

Tipton, M.J., Golden, F.S., "A proposed decision-making guide for the search, rescue and resuscitation of submersion (head under) victims based on expert opinion", *Resuscitation* 2011, 82, 819–824

Tipton M.J., et al., "Immersion deaths and deterioration in swimming performance in cold water", *Lancet*, 1999 Aug 21

Tipton, M.J., et al., "Cold water immersion: kill or cure?", *Exp Physiol*, 2017 Nov

Waag, T., Hesselberg, O., Reinertsen, R.E., "Heat Production During Cold Water Immersion: The Role of Shivering and Exercise in the Development of Hypothermia", *Arct. Med. Res.*, 1995, 54 (Suppl. S2), pp. 60–64

World Health Organization – https://www.who.int/news-room/fact-sheets/detail/drowning

www.telegraph.co.uk/topics/christmas/9719063/The-swimmers-with-ice-in-their-veins.htm (accessed 27 April 2021)

https://hjerteforeningen.dk/2017/02/vinterbadning-vaen-langsomt-kroppen-chokket/

www.badevand.dk

www.respektforvand.dk

Chapter 10

Brenke, R., "Winter swimming – An extreme form of body hardening", *Therapeutikon* 1990, 4, 466–472

Collier, N., Massey, H., Lomax, M., Harper, M., Tipton, M., "Habitual cold water swimming and upper respiratory tract infection", *Extrem. Physiol. Med.* 2015, 4, A36

Cypess, A.M., Weiner, L.S., Roberts-Toler, C., Elía, E.F., Kessler, S.H., Kahn, P.A., English, J., Chatman, K., Trauger, S.A., Doria, A., et al., (2015) "Activation of Human Brown Adipose Tissue by a β3-Adrenergic Receptor Agonist", *Cell Metab*, 21, 33–38

Dhabhar, F.S., "Effects of stress on immune function: The good, the bad, and the beautiful" *Immunol. Res.*, 2014, 58, 193–210

Dugué, B., Leppänen, E. "Adaptation related to cytokines in man: effects of regular swimming in ice-cold water", *Clin Physiol.* 2000 Mar; 20(2):114-21

Dulac, S., Quirion, A., DeCarufel, D., LeBlanc, J., Jobin, M., Côte, J., Brisson, G.R., Lavoie, J.M., Diamond, P., "Metabolic and hormonal responses to long-distance swimming in cold water", *Int. J. Sports Med.*, 1987, 8, 352–356

Freedman, et al., "Arterial and Venous Thrombosis", *Harrison's Principles of Internal Medicine*, 20th edition (New York, NY: McGraw-Hill, 2018)

Gibas-Dorna, M., et al., "Cold Water Swimming Beneficially Modulates Insulin Sensitivity in Middle-Aged Individuals", 2016. 24(4): pp. 547–554

Gibas-Dorna M., et al., "Variations in leptin and insulin levels within one swimming season in non-obese female cold water swimmers" *Scand J Clin Lab Invest.*, 2016

Gundle, L., Atkinson, A., "Pregnancy, cold water swimming and cortisol: The effect of cold water swimming on obstetric outcomes", *Med. Hypotheses* 2020, 144, 109977

Hansson, G.K., "Inflammation, atherosclerosis, and coronary artery disease" *N Engl J Med.*, 2005, Apr 21 Review

Hanssen, M.J.W., Hoeks, J., Brans, B., van der Lans, A.A.J.J., Schaart, G., van den Driessche, J.J., Jörgensen, J.A., Boekschoten, M.V., Hesselink, M.K.C., Havekes, B., et al., (2015) "Short-term cold acclimation improves insulin sensitivity in patients with type 2 diabetes mellitus", *Nat. Med.* 21, 6–10

Hanssen, M.J.W., Van Der Lans, A.A.J.J., Brans, B., Hoeks, J., Jardon, K.M.C., Schaart, G., Mottaghy, F.M., Schrauwen, P., and Van Marken Lichtenbelt, W.D., (2016) "Short-term cold acclimation recruits brown adipose tissue in obese humans", *Diabetes* 65, 1179–1189

Hartwig, A.C. "Peripheral beta-endorphin and pain modulation", *Anesth Prog.*, 1991, Review

Heinonen, I., et al., "Effects of heat and cold on health, with special reference to Finnish sauna bathing", *Am J Physiol Regul Integr Comp Physiol.*, 2018 May 1

Hermanussen, M., Jensen, F., Hirsch, N., Friedel, K., Kröger, B., Lang, R., Just, S., Ulmer, J., Schaff, M., Ahnert, P., "Acute and chronic effects of winter swimming on LH, FSH, prolactin, growth hormone, TSH, Cortisol, serum glucose and insulin", *Arct. Med. Res.* 1995, 54, 45–51

Hirotsu, C., Tufik, S., and Andersen, M.L., (2015) "Interactions between sleep, stress, and metabolism: From physiological to pathological conditions", *Sleep Sci.* 8, 143–152

Huttunen P, et al., "Winter swimming improves general well-being", *Int J Circumpolar Health*, 2004 May

Huttunen, P., Lando, N.G., Meshtsheryakov, V.A., Lyutov, V.A., "Effects of long-distance swimming in cold water on temperature, blood pressure and stress hormones in winter swimmers", *J. Therm. Biol.* 2000, 25, 171–174

Huttunen, P., Rintamäki, H., Hirvonen, J., "Effect of regular winter swimming on the activity of the sympathoadrenal system before and after a single cold water immersion", *Int. J. Circumpolar Health*, 2001, 60, 400–406

Kauppinen, K., Pajari-Backas, M., Volin, P., Vakkuri, O., "Some endocrine responses to sauna, shower and ice water immersion", *Arct. Med. Res.*, 1989, 48, 131–139

Knechtle, B., Stjepanovic, M., Knechtle, C., Rosemann, T., Sousa, C.V., Nikolaidis, P.T., "Physiological Responses to Swimming Repetitive 'Ice Miles'", *J. Strength Cond. Res.*, 2020

Kolettis, T.M., Kolettis, M.T., "Winter swimming: Healthy or hazardous? Evidence and hypotheses", *Med. Hypotheses* 2003, 61, 654–656

Johnson, D.G., Hayward, J.S., Jacobs, T.P., Collis, M.L., Eckerson, J.D., Williams, R.H., "Plasma norepinephrine responses of man in cold water", *J. Appl. Physiol. Respir. Environ. Exerc. Physiol.*, 1977, 43, 216–220

Lee, P., Smith, S., Linderman, J., Courville, A.B., Brychta, R.J., Dieckmann, W., Werner, C.D., Chen, K.Y., and Celi, F.S., (2014) "Temperature-Acclimated Brown Adipose Tissue Modulates Insulin Sensitivity in Humans", *Diabetes* 63, 3686–3698

Levine, J.A., "Non-exercise activity thermogenesis (NEAT)", *Best Pract Res Clin Endocrinol Metab.*, 2002 Dec. Review

Lubkowska A. et al., "Winter-swimming as a building-up body resistance factor inducing adaptive changes in the oxidant/ antioxidant status", *Scand J Clin Lab Invest.* 2013

O'Mara, A.E., Johnson, J.W., Linderman, J.D., Brychta, R.J., McGehee, S., Fletcher, L.A., Fink, Y.A., Kapuria, D., Cassimatis, T.M., Kelsey, N., et al., (2020) "Chronic mirabegron treatment increases human brown fat, HDL cholesterol and insulin sensitivity", *J. Clin. Invest.* 130

Päth, G., Scherbaum, W.A., and Bornstein, S.R., (2000) "The role of interleukin-6 in the human adrenal gland", *Eur. J. Clin. Invest.*, 30, 91–95

Redwine, L., Hauger, R.L., Gillin, J.C., and Irwin, M., (2000) "Effects of Sleep and Sleep Deprivation on Interleukin-6, Growth Hormone, Cortisol and Melatonin Levels in Humans", 1. *J. Clin. Endocrinol. Metab.*, 85, 3597–3603

Sirgy, M.J., "Positive balance: a hierarchical perspective of positive mental health", *Qual Life Res.* 2019 Jul; 282

Siems, W.G., et al., "Improved antioxidative protection in winter swimmers", *QJM.* 1999 Apr

Tanaka, H., et al., "Arterial stiffness of lifelong Japanese female pearl divers", *Am J Physiol Regul Integr Comp Physiol.* 2016 May

Tipton, M.J., et al., "Cold water immersion: kill or cure?", *Exp Physiol.*, 2017 Nov

Valko, M, et al., "Free radicals and antioxidants in normal physiological functions and human disease", *Int J Biochem Cell Biol.*, 2007

Van Tulleken, C., Tipton, M., Massey, H., Harper, C.M., "Open water swimming as a treatment for major depressive disorder", *BMJ Case Rep.*, 2018

Vybiral, S. et al., "Thermoregulation in winter swimmers and physiological significance of human catecholamine thermogenesis", *Exp Physiol* 2000

Zenner, R., De Decker, D., Clement, D., "Blood-pressure response to swimming in ice-cold water", *Lancet*, 1980, 315, 120–121

Chapter 11

Eckel, Robert H., "The Metabolic Syndrome", *Harrison's Principles of Internal Medicine*, 20th edition (New York, NY: McGraw-Hill, 2018)

Flier, et al., "Pathobiology of Obesity", *Harrison's Principles of Internal Medicine*, 20th edition (New York, NY: McGraw-Hill, 2018)

Friedman J., "20 years of leptin: leptin at 20:

an overview", *J Endocrinol.*, 2014 Aug 13. Review

Gibas-Dorna, M., et al., "Cold Water Swimming Beneficially Modulates Insulin Sensitivity in Middle-Aged Individuals", *J Aging Phys Act*, 2016, 24(4): pp. 547–554

Gibas-Dorna, M., et al., "Variations in leptin and insulin levels within one swimming season in non-obese female cold water swimmers", *Scand J Clin Lab Invest.*, 2016

Johnson F., et al., "Could increased time spent in a thermal comfort zone contribute to population increases in obesity?", *Obes Rev.*, 2011 July

Ouellet, V., et al., "Outdoor temperature, age, sex, body mass index and diabetic status determine the prevalence, mass and glucose-uptake activity of 18F-FDG-detected BAT in humans", *J Clin Endocrinol Metab*, 2011

Pasricha, P.J., "Hunger games: is your stomach making you fat?", *Gastroenterology*, 2015 Mar

Søberg S., et al., "FGF21 Is a Sugar-Induced Hormone Associated with Sweet Intake and Preference in Humans", *Cell Metab.*, 2017 May 2

Søberg S., et al., "FGF21, a liver hormone that inhibits alcohol intake in mice, increases in human circulation after acute alcohol ingestion and sustained binge drinking at Oktoberfest", *Mol Metab.*, 2018 May

Turner, J.B., et al., "The effects of indoor and outdoor temperature on metabolic rate and adipose tissue – the Mississippi perspective on the obesity epidemic", *Rev Endocr Metab Disord.*, 2016 Mar

Chapter 12

Gelenberg, A.J. et al., "Assessing and treating depression in primary care medicine", *Am J Med*, 2007

Hartwig, A.C., "Peripheral beta-endorphin and pain modulation", *Anesth Prog.*, 1991, Review

Jansky, L., et al., "Change in sympathetic activity, cardiovascular functions and plasma hormone concentrations due to cold water immersion in men", *Eur J Appl Physiol Occup Physiol*, 1996

Jedema, H.P., et al., "Chronic cold exposure potentiates CRH-evoked increases in electrophysiologic activity of locus coeruleus neurons", *Biol Psy*, 2001

Jones, D.M., et al., "Cold acclimation and

cognitive performance: A review", *Auton Neurosci*, 2017 Dec

Messing, Robert O., et al., "Biology of Psychiatric Disorders", *Harrison's Principles of Internal Medicine*, 20th edition (New York, NY: McGraw-Hill, 2018)

Miller, A.H., et al., "The role of inflammation in depression: from evolutionary imperative to modern treatment target", *Nat Rev Immunol*, 2016

Nutt, D.J., "The neuropharmacology of serotonin and noradrenaline in depression", *Int Clin Psychopharmacol*, 2002

Sirgy, M.J., "Positive balance: a hierarchical perspective of positive mental health", *Qual Life Res.*, 2019 Jul

Van Tulleken, C. et al., "Open water swimming as a treatment for major depressive disorder", *BMJ Case Rep.*, 2018 Aug

Vaswani, K.K. et al., "Cold swim stress induced changes in the levels of opioid peptides in the rat CNS and peripheral tissues", *Pharmacol Biochem Behav*, 1988

Webb, T.L., et al., "Using theories of behaviour change to inform interventions for addictive behaviours", *Addiction*, 2010 Nov

https://www.who.int/mental_health/management/depression/wfmh_paper_depression_wmhd_2012.pdf

Chapter 13

Baker, Lindsay B., "Physiology of sweat gland function: The roles of sweating and sweat composition in human health", *Temperature*, 2019, 211–259, 6(3)

Costa, R.J.S., et al., (2014) "Heat acclimation responses of an ultra-endurance running group preparing for hot desert-based competition", *Eur. J. Sport Sci.*, 14

Cox, N.J., et al., "Sauna to transiently improve pulmonary function in patients with obstructive lung disease", *Arch Phys Med Rehabil.*, 1989; 70(13): 911–913

Crinnion, Walter, "Components of practical clinical detox programs – sauna as a therapeutic tool", *Altern Ther Health Med*, Mar-Apr 2007; 13(2): 154-156

Ernst, E., et al., "Regular sauna bathing and the incidence of common colds", Ann Med. 1990; 22(4): 225–227

Filingeri, D., Zhang, H., and Arens, E.A., (2017) "Characteristics of the local

cutaneous sensory thermoneutral zone",
J. Neurophysiol. 117, 1797–1806 Fox, R.H.,
et al., "A thermoregulatory function test
using controlled hyperthermia", *J Appl
Physiol* 23: 267–275, 1967

Gagge, A.P., and Gonzalez, R.R., (2011)
"Mechanisms of Heat Exchange:
Biophysics and Physiology",
Comprehensive Physiology (Hoboken,
NJ, USA: John Wiley & Sons, Inc.),
pp. 45–84

Gryka, D., et al., "The effect of sauna bathing
on lipid profile in young, physically active,
male subjects". *Int J Occup Med Environ
Health*, 2014 Aug; 27

Hargreaves, M., (2008) "Physiological limits
to exercise performance in the heat",
*Journal of Science and Medicine in Sport/
Sports Medicine Australia*, 11(1), 6671

Hong, S. K. et al., "Peripheral blood flow
and heat flux of Korean women divers",
Federation Proceedings, 1969, 1143–1148,
28(3)

Hussain, J.N., et al., "A hot topic for health:
Results of the Global Sauna Survey",
Complement Ther Med., 2019 Jun

Iggo A, et al., "Impulse coding in primate
cutaneous thermoreceptors in dynamic
thermal conditions", *J Physiol*, 1971

Janssent, Clemens W., et al., "Whole-Body
Hyperthermia for the Treatment of Major
Depressive Disorder – A Randomized
Clinical Trial", *JAMA Psychiatry*, 2016;
73(8): 789–795

Köteles, F., et al., "Inhaled peppermint,
rosemary and eucalyptus essential oils
do not change spirometry in healthy
individuals", *Physiol Behav.*, 2018 Oct

Kunutsor, S.K., et al., "Sauna bathing reduces
the risk of stroke in Finnish men and
women: a prospective cohort study",
Neurology, 2018 May

Kunutsor, S.K., et al., "Sauna bathing reduces
the risk of venous thromboembolism:
a prospective cohort study", *Eur J
Epidemiol*, 2019 Aug 1

Kunutsor, S.K., et al., "Frequent sauna
bathing may reduce the risk of
pneumonia in middle-aged Caucasian
men: The KIHD prospective cohort
study", *Respir Med.*, 2017 Nov

Kunutsor, S.K., Laukkanen, T., Laukkanen,
J.A., "Sauna bathing reduces the risk
of respiratory diseases: a long-term
prospective cohort study", *Eur J
Epidemiol.* 2017; 32(12):1107–1111

Laatikainen, T., et al., "Response of plasma
endorphins, prolactin and catecholamines
in women to intense heat in a sauna",
*European Journal of Applied Physiology
and Occupational Physiology*, 1988,
98–102, 57(1)

Laitinen, L.A., et al., "Lungs and ventilation
in sauna", *Ann Clin Res.*, 1988

Laukkanen, J.A., et al., "Is sauna bathing
protective of sudden cardiac death? A
review of the evidence", *Prog Cardiovasc
Dis.*, 2019 May 2019, Review

Laukkanen, J.A., et al., "Cardiovascular and
Other Health Benefits of Sauna Bathing:
A Review of the Evidence", *Mayo Clin
Proc.*, 2018 Aug

Laukkanen, J.A., et al., "Combined Effect
of Sauna Bathing and Cardiorespiratory
Fitness on the Risk of Sudden Cardiac
Deaths in Caucasian Men: A Long-
term Prospective Cohort Study", *Prog
Cardiovasc Dis.*, 2018

Laukkanen T, et al., "Sauna Bathing and Risk
of Psychotic Disorders: A Prospective
Cohort Study", *Med Princ Pract.*, 2018;
27(6): 562–569

Laukkanen. T., et al., "Association between
sauna bathing and fatal cardiovascular
and all-cause mortality events", *JAMA
Intern Med.*, 2015

Laukkanen T., et al., "Sauna bathing is
inversely associated with dementia and
Alzheimer's disease in middle-aged
Finnish men", *Age Ageing*, 2017 Mar

Magalhaes, F.C., et al., (2010)
"Thermoregulatory efficiency is increased
after heat acclimation in tropical natives",
Journal of Physiological Anthropology,
29(1), 112

Narita, M., Khotib, J., Suzuki, M., Ozaki, S.,
Yajima, Y., and Suzuki, T., "Heterologous
mu-opioid receptor adaptation by
repeated stimulation of kappa-opioid
receptor: up-regulation of G-protein
activation and antinociception", J.
Neurochem, 85, no. 5 (June 2003): 1171–1179

Patterson, M.J., Stocks, J.M., Taylor, N.A.S.,
"Humid heat acclimation does not elicit a
preferential sweat redistribution towards
the limbs", *Am J Physiol* 286: R512–R518,
2004

Petrofsky, J.S. "Resting blood flow in
the skin: does it exist, and what is the
influence of temperature, aging and

diabetes?", *J Diabetes Sci Technol.*, 2012 May, Review

Pilch, W., "Comparison of physiological reactions and physiological strain in healthy men under heat stress in dry and steam heat saunas", *Biol Sport*, 2014 Jun; 31(2): 145-149. doi: 0.5604/20831862.1099045, Epub 2014 Apr 5

Vescovi, P.P., Casti, A., Michelini, M., Maninetti, L., Pedrazzoni, M. and Passeri., M., "Plasma ACTH, beta-endorphin, prolactin, growth hormone and luteinizing hormone levels after thermal stress, heat and cold", *Stress Medicine* 8, no. 3 (July 1992): 187-91. doi: 10.1002/smi.2460080310

Woodworth, R.S., et al., "Experimental psychology", (New York: Holt, Rinehart and Winston, 1965)

WHO., Revised global burden of disease 2002 estimates. 2004. http://www.who.int/healthinfo/global_ burden_disease/estimates_regional_2002_ revised/en/ (set 1. October 2019).

PICTURE CREDITS

Alamy: Front endpaper Alan Dawson; 6 Keith Morris News; 9, 31, 145, 205 dpa; 11, 67 Helena Wahlman; 14 steeve-x-art; 16 Walker Art Library; 18 Science History Images; 19 Süddeutsche Zeitung Photo; 24, 170 C12; 27, 132, 178, 215 Johner Images; 28, 140 Michele Ursi; 38 A. Howden – Australia Stock Photography; 41 Alexander Cvetkov; 42 Christian Kober; 45, 222 Sergi Reboredo; 46, 109, 125 ZUMA Press; 48, 92 Andrey Nekrasov; 50 Aly Song; 52 Simon Dack News; 56 Barry Lewis; 61 David Buzzard; 64-65 Yuri Maltsev; 70-71, 160 Maciej Bledowski; 74 rangizzz; 77 Sergey Fayzulin; 81 Santosh Chavan; 83 Mint Images; 84 Nikolay Vinokurov; 89 Aleksandr Volkov; 95 Vova Pomortzeff; 97, 120-121 David W. Cerny; 100 Seiji Oka; 105 Emma Stoner; 110 Zoonar/Maxim Petrichuk; 118 Mathieu B. Morin; 122 Zivica Kerkez; 127 Seppo Hinkula; 128-129 Troika; 138 Dominic Dibbs; 141 Dominic Lipinski/PA Images; 142 Keith Larby; 149 Nick Savage; 150, 163, 198-199 Ragnar Th. Sigurdsson; 157 Else M. Lundal; 159 Viktor Yatsuk; 167 REUTERS; 172 ITAR-TASS News Agency; 185 Vladimir Pomortzeff; 187 Toby Melville; 192-193 Jean Schweitzer; 210 Vladislav Zadjko; 220 Lauri Rotko; 225 Petri Jauhianen; 226-227 Ints Kalnins; 235 Michael Sheridan; 240-241 Natalia Golubnycha.

Peter Bradley (author of *Waterproof – Winter Swimmers of Brockwell Park Lido*): 148.

Getty Images: 20 E. Dean/Hulton Archive; 21 James L. Amos/Corbis.

iStock: 43 nemar74; 63 GAPS.

Lars Kruse: 256.

Shutterstock: Back endpaper Raland; 2 Dudarev Mikhail; 32 Michele Ursi; 35 Inga Gedrovicha; 69 deniska_ua; 116 LidiaSpirina; 123 LDarin; 130 NZ3; 154 Eric Isselee; 165 ilmarinfoto; 180 Jevgenijs Skolokovs; 189 Halfpoint; 195 4H4 Photography; 202 Kzenon; 206 Tramp57; 217 Yanya; 228 Stocklite; 238 Hvoenok.

Susanna Søberg: 247.

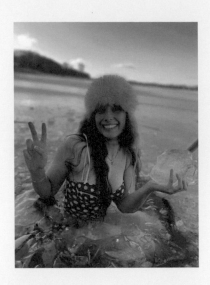

DR SUSANNA SØBERG earned her PhD researching metabolism and has worked for many years designing and conducting clinical studies. Her most recent research and the background for this book have been on fat reduction through winter swimming at the Tryg Foundation's Centre for Physical Activity, Denmark. *Winter Swimming*, to be published in more than thirteen languages, is her first book.

DR ELIZABETH DENOMA is a freelance editor, translator and publishing consultant with a PhD in Scandinavian languages and literature from the University of Washington. She's worked at University of Washington, University of Wisconsin, Microsoft, Websters Multimedia Publishing and most recently at Amazon Crossing as a Senior Editor acquiring and editing global literature for translation into English.

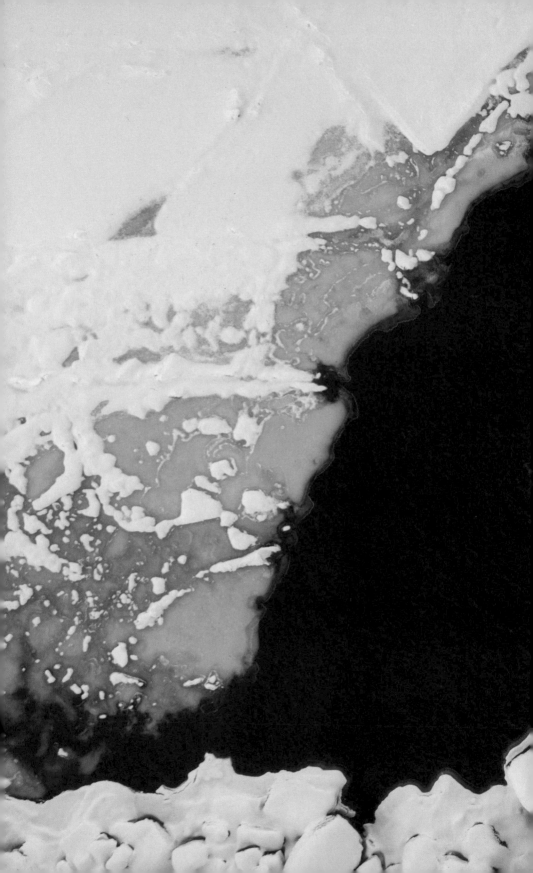